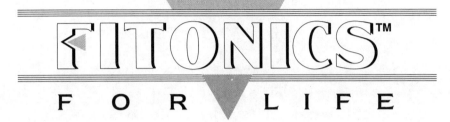

FITONICS™

FOR LIFE

Other Books by Marilyn Diamond

FIT FOR LIFE
FIT FOR LIFE II
THE AMERICAN VEGETARIAN COOKBOOK
A NEW WAY OF EATING FROM FIT FOR LIFE

FITONICS™

FOR LIFE

Marilyn Diamond
AND
Dr. Donald Burton Schnell

Exercise Illustrations by Mona Mark

AVON BOOKS ◢◣ NEW YORK

| VISIT OUR WEBSITE AT |
| http://Avon Books.com |

FITONICS™ FOR LIFE is an original publication of Avon Books.
This work has never before appeared in book form.

AVON BOOKS
A division of
The Hearst Corporation
1350 Avenue of the Americas
New York, New York 10019

Copyright © 1996 by FITONICS INC.
Illustrations copyright © 1996 by Mona Mark
Text design by Stanley S. Drate/Folio Graphics Co. Inc.
Published by arrangement with FITONICS INC.
Library of Congress Catalog Card Number: 96-22815
ISBN: 0-380-97389-8

Library of Congress Cataloging in Publication Data:
Diamond, Marilyn.
Fitonics for life / Marilyn Diamond and Donald Burton Schnell.
p. cm.
Includes bibliographical references and index.
1. Weight loss. 2. Reducing diets. 3. Reducing exercises.
I. Schnell, Donald Burton. II. Title.
RM222.2.D484 1996 96-22815
613.2'5—dc20 CIP

First Avon Books Hardcover Printing: December 1996

AVON TRADEMARK REG. U.S. PAT. OFF. AND IN OTHER COUNTRIES, MARCA REGISTRADA, HECHO EN U.S.A.

Printed in the U.S.A.

FIRST EDITION

OPM 10 9 8 7 6 5 4 3 2 1

In Memoriam

To our dearly departed friend,
Bob Goodman,
who joyously worked to bring
FITONICS nutritional products to our readers.
We will miss you.

*This book is dedicated to all the loyal FIT FOR LIFE fans
and supporters who, over the years, have shared their
successes and inspired FITONICS . . .*

*to our beloved children, Greg, Lisa, Beau and Michael,
their dreams of the future give us no choice but to strive
for a better world . . .*

*to our dear parents, Fran and Bernie Horecker and Jim and
Ginger Schnell, and Dena Winn, whose love and
enthusiastic support we will always cherish . . .*

*to Cindy, who delivered the message of the angels and
brought us together . . .*

*to Grandma Ida, who at age ninety-five felt our love and
gave her blessing . . .*

and to you, dear reader . . .

may your life, through this book, forever, be enriched.

▼

Acknowledgments

▼

We wish to express our love and gratitude:

To Mel Berger at the William Morris Agency, for wholeheartedly championing the FITONICS project; Marcy Posner, for reaching out across the oceans; and Claudia Cross, for cheerfully lending assistance.

To Lisa Neuwirth, for her fabulous recipes and tireless dedication to the FITONICS mission.

To Janet Allen, for being willing to be our liaison to the world, assuming any task, any time, any place, far beyond the call of duty.

To the dedicated staff at Avon Books:

Michael Weinstein and Lou Aronica, for believing in our work; Darlene DeLillo, for listening and helping to package the message; Christine Zika, for her passion and enthusiasm in editing; Jennifer Hershey, for the excellent hands-on effort in the final editing process; Anne Marie Spagnuolo, for helping pull it all together; Debby Tobias, for being head cheerleader; Joan Schulhafer and Laura Mullen, for spreading the word; and Tom Egner, for his brilliant design of the cover.

To our family and extended family:

Charles and Mary Lynn Goldstein, for being the doting aunt and uncle; Linda and Brendan Lally, for offering support when it was so needed; James Schnell, for handling the mail with so much heart; James McCrary and Rick Cahill, our Center leaders, always there for us selflessly whenever we call; Nels Gullerud and Pete Buccholtz, for the undemanding and unconditional love they always flow in our direction; and Frank Renner, for his prayers.

To the many excellent professionals who supported us to do our work:

Michael J. Glass, for his loyalty and integrity; John Anderson at Global Nutrition, for making the effort to help us bring the finest nutritional support to our readers; Tina Cherie and Kay Berry at Saks Fifth Avenue, for tirelessly shaping the image; and Seymour Sacks, for believing in us.

And with deepest love and respect, our homage:

To Victor Kulvinskas, for inspiring the enzyme story; Jack LaLanne, for carrying the torch and setting the example; and, most of all:

To the Great Almighty, who sent us all of the above, along with Angel, to do the purring.

Contents

PART TWO

▼

BREAKTHROUGH THINKING

PART THREE

▼

THE DAILY EXERCISE BREAKTHROUGH

PART FOUR

▼

THE FITONICS FORMULA FOR
HIGH-ENERGY EATING

PART FIVE

▼

FITONICS RECIPES FOR LIFE!

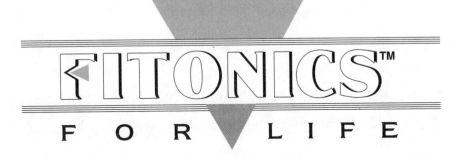

FITONICS™
F O R L I F E

Fit: Wellness in mind, body, and spirit.

Tonics: Substances, or ideas, that invigorate or strengthen by acting as stimulants or by gradually restoring health.

▼
Let's Go Forward!
▼

FIT FOR LIFE came on the American weight-loss scene in June of 1985. It was a time not unlike what we are experiencing today—a time in which Americans were clamoring for new dietary solutions. As a population, we were confused, out of energy, and bored to death with calorie counting, measured portions, and the endless litany of ineffective diets that would come and go without lasting results. After a lifetime of interest in food, science, and medicine, and over a decade of research on the FIT FOR LIFE program, I felt a calling to answer the public demand for new and relevant information.

The book I co-authored as a result proved itself to be right on target. *FIT FOR LIFE* made its appearance on the *New York Times* Bestseller List within weeks of its publication, barreled into the #1 position, and held it . . . for an unprecedented *forty* weeks. Within months, it became Warner Books's first million-selling hardcover, breaking every record for its time. After ninety weeks on the bestseller list, it was rated the #1 diet and health book in publishing history. It appeared along with *Gone With the Wind* and the Bible on the *Publishers Weekly* list of the top twenty-five bestselling books ever written.

During the decade that followed, *FIT FOR LIFE* was translated into over thirty languages and reached bestseller status around the world—in Germany, Canada, Sweden, Australia, South Africa, and Israel, to give only a partial list. Worldwide sales now hover at around ten million copies.

As you can imagine, all of this completely changed my life. I felt a deep connection to the readers of all ages and from all

1

walks of life for whom the program was working so well. Each day, I thanked God for the blessing and the opportunity to be of assistance to so many people.

As the demand for additional support grew, I went back to "the drawing board," revised my first book, *A NEW WAY OF EATING FROM FIT FOR LIFE*, written in 1978, co-authored *FIT FOR LIFE II*, and authored the encyclopedic *AMERICAN VEGE-TARIAN COOKBOOK FROM THE FIT FOR LIFE KITCHEN*. In 1990, a market research survey found that for every one of the ten million copies purchased, five people were introduced to the program. With *fifty million* lives touched, no other health and weight-loss program in history can claim such significant multinational and demographic tests of success.

The Beginnings of a Movement

The principles of *FIT FOR LIFE* are still relevant today. Wherever I go, I hear inspiring stories of continued success. Having put weight, energy, and digestive problems behind them, *FIT FOR LIFE* enthusiasts ranging in age from fifteen to ninety-five are literally a force of converts and missionaries. Nearly one thousand testimonial letters a month from grateful readers still flood our mailroom.

Read what Richard Clark George from Angwin, California, wrote in May 1995, and judge yourself:

"I owe my life to your program. Through faith in God and following your guidelines for nutritional and healthful living, I lost 155 pounds in one year and two months. [Prior to that time,] I was terribly depressed, and my gallbladder became infected with stones as a result. On December 22, 1992, I entered a local hospital to have the gallbladder removed surgically. Because of a mistake made by a nurse who administerd my anesthesia, I almost died on the operating table. They spent thirty minutes bringing me back to life; it was only through

the grace of God that I survived. After a successful 5½-hour surgery on January 7, 1993, I began to implement your program. By the spring of 1994, I weighed about 170.

"[Before,] I was lonely, obese, and had no hope for the future. Now I am close friends with a beautiful Russian woman (whom I am considering marrying someday). I am in your debt for the rest of my life."

In January 1996, Jim Jensen from West Jordan, Utah, wrote:

"In November of 1992 a friend of mine introduced me to your book, FIT FOR LIFE. The book made it sound like sensible eating and fitness could easily be mastered. Since I've had a weight problem my entire life (I weighed close to 400 lbs. at this point) I couldn't believe it could be that easy, so I had to give it a try.

"I read your book and started to apply your eating habits to my daily life. I started with fresh fruit in the morning, salad for lunch, and 'normal' dinner. You never told me I couldn't have anything like so many other diets do.

"In January of 1993 I started adding exercise to my program. I started walking or riding a bike for twenty minutes a day. The weight started to peel off at this point. Within months I was walking or running anywhere between thirty and ninety minutes a day and loving it!

"I now weigh in between 195 and 200 lbs. I've maintained this weight since September 1993 and I know I can do this for the rest of my life. I love the feeling of being in control of my weight. I have energy and good health. I have clothes that fit me off the rack; no more shopping in 'big man' stores. When I see people I haven't seen in a long while in the street, they don't even recognize me. You started me on the road to good health, and I plan to continue down that road using the tools you have provided."

Finally, from Dale and Peggy Free of Cincinnati, Ohio, in February 1995:

"We would like to thank you for your FIT FOR LIFE program. Since last May, Dale has lost 65 pounds, and Peggy has lost nearly 50. After ten months of following the program, we feel like we've made a lifetime commitment. We were concerned about maintenance after we lost the weight. We think we've found the answer now with your AMERICAN VEGETARIAN COOKBOOK. It was just what we need to keep from being bored with our meals. Since losing the weight, we've been able to get back into a running routine. Now, at ages 57 and 52, the exercise is easier than ever."

The letters and personal interviews over the years have made all the hard work and demanding schedules worth every minute of effort. Readers, having tasted the benefits of health from *FIT FOR LIFE*, developed voracious appetites . . . for more information! Many were seeking to reach for their highest health potential. *And so was I!*

The Next Step

In the decade since 1985, I have undergone a dramatic evolution. The changes in my life have been all-encompassing, affecting my personal life, my business associations, and the very foundation of my approach toward living. In 1992 I experienced the wondrous blessing that even as I brought the FIT FOR LIFE phase of my life to an end, a more positive expression of my ideas began to manifest itself. At that time, I was fully aware that after helping millions of people lose millions of pounds of excess weight, I was going to do it again—and in an even more effective way.

On July 30, 1992, I attended a unique meditation intensive led by clinical hypnotherapist Dr. Donald Burton Schnell. Dr. Schnell is the originator of HYPNO-MEDITATION™, an effective synthesis of Western and Eastern spiritual teachings and techniques. Expecting simply to experience just one more of the dozens of meditation workshops I had attended, I was surprised to find myself in the presence of a deeply evolved, broadly educated specialist in Natural Health, including diet, supplementation, and exercise to lose weight, all choices that lead to spiritual evolution and better health. Here was clearly a master at Natural Health, my field of expertise for over twenty years.

At the intensive and the many others that followed, I began to experience a profound regeneration. In one particular meditation session, accessing the super-conscious, I clearly saw myself, dressed in flowing white, rising up from the darkness, my hands above my head, tears of joy streaming from my eyes, my face reflecting a radiance and happiness I had not felt for many years. As I reached toward the heavens, cinder blocks and bars were tumbling and crashing around me. I knew at that moment a new life for me had started to unfold. The spiritual energy igniting my being was transforming everything. When those who knew me complimented me on my rejuvenation, I found myself sharing happily, "What I have found is even better than fruit in the morning!"

Later that year, I had the opportunity to travel with Dr. Schnell to India, where he introduced me to some of the great Eastern spiritual masters with whom he had studied meditation over the years. Plunged in healing meditation for hours every day, undergoing one of the pivotal spiritual experiences of my life, I connected to the essential energy that would begin to propel me to create a new and updated lifestyle program of physical, mental, and spiritual balance—one that would reflect not only the health and fitness of the body but also the radiance of the soul. It was after one unusually deep meditation that Dr. Schnell proposed "FITONICS" as the name of a new health movement that he believed—as did I—the West sorely needed. That trip to India, for me, was the beginning of my FITONICS adventure with Donald Schnell.

A Clean Slate

For nearly a year following that trip, I wiped the slate clean of dietary principles I had lived by for two decades. I was eager to test the dietary theories of others, *and* my own, and I knew the best way to ascertain what would be most truly effective for this era would be to return myself to an "average" state of health, and then begin anew.

Some of my readers may be surprised to hear that, after twenty years of vegetarian eating, and the authoring of two vegetarian cookbooks, I began the research for FITONICS by sitting down to a cheeseburger, french fries, and a *diet soda*! Although for years I had been walking three or four miles—three times a week—and had my own yoga routine, I stopped exercising regularly. What I was attempting to do was revisit, firsthand, the effects of today's junkier-than-ever Standard American Diet (S.A.D.) and more-sedentary-than-ever mainstream lifestyle.

I must admit, sometimes the experiment was quite enjoyable. I had become so strict in my diet over the years—far stricter than the mandates in *FIT FOR LIFE*—that I almost never dined out, unless it was at a health food restaurant. Instead, for eighteen years, I had been spending six to eight hours in the kitchen every day, preparing food for my writings and my family. Now Donald seized the opportunity, saying, "This will be fun! You deserve a break. Let me take you out dining and dancing."

I bought a whole new wardrobe of evening clothes. We ate in the finest restaurants in town, multicourse meals of foods I had loved as a young woman living in Paris and traveling throughout Europe. I had wine with my meals and ate desserts I thought I had forsaken for the rest of my life.

Within a few months, I had gained fat on my thighs and around my middle, my energy level sank, and my stomach frequently hurt! Even more telling was that I was suddenly painfully conscious of my vulnerability to disease. For the first and only time in my life, I began to experience hot flashes and the roller-coaster mood swings that accompany hormonal shifts. I went from being truly confident that my health was in my control to fearing cancer and heart disease. I began to take over-the-counter drugs, sought traditional medical attention, and found myself at night—when I should have been sleeping—lying awake and worrying about the subtle symptoms of degeneration that my lifestyle was causing. Meditation and peaceful reflection became difficult, if not impossible, and my focus—as I became nutritionally deficient—turned more and more toward frequent meals and sweets.

With a weight gain nearing *twenty* pounds, I had deliberately allowed myself to experience what the largest portion of our population feels every minute of every day. From firsthand experience I can now confirm that we truly are what we eat, and we have the choice to eat food that will *empower* or destroy us. What I experienced firsthand was that when we eat "fast" food, we begin to die faster. If we eat "junk," our lives begin to lose the quality that good health assures us.

Now, when I advocate sensible changes in lifestyle and swearing off poisonous American fast food, I do it from a deeper level of empathy than ever before.

How Did I Put Myself
Back in Shape?

With Donald Schnell as my partner, I began a period of research that brought me over a year's time to the FITONICS program.

▶ I signed on with several personal trainers, wishing to experience a broad example of weight training, body building, and the diets that frequently are recommended to accompany that approach. I tried the high-protein weight-lifters' *anabolic* diet, the forerunner of THE ZONE, and found myself constipated, with bad breath and a subtle *heavy-hearted* feeling. Although I did build muscle, there was still too much fat on my body for my taste. I also felt that even a once or twice weekly visit to a personal trainer was far too expensive and didn't dovetail with my natural health philosophy. After all, how many of us can manage the financial and time commitment required from a personal trainer?

▶ I cut out all protein and went on a high-carbohydrate diet, adding demanding aerobics to my life. What a surprise to find myself once again feeling heavy and a bit lethargic, with a subtle and continuous hunger. Although I bicycled and used the treadmill incessantly, my thighs remained doughy and Donald fought to no avail to lose weight he had gained at his waist.

▶ I went to a final extreme, with a three-week visit to the Hippocrates Health Institute in West Palm Beach, Florida, directed by Natural Health pioneers Brian and Anna Marie Clement.[1] At Hippocrates, a raw-food healing center, no fruit but watermelon juice is allowed, and instead quantities of sprouts, green juices, raw sauerkraut, sea vegetables, garlic, and salads are served twice a day.

As Donald and I lost fat and inches (and some of the muscle we had both built), we saw our skin and eyes begin to glow on this well-prepared and well-researched program, and we witnessed other program participants learn the tools for healing life-threatening maladies using this *natural* healing regimen. It was an inspiring experience, and it was also clear that such a strategy would also be very challenging to implement in one's own home. But elements of what I learned there will always stay with me.

---

[1]Brian R. Clement. *Living Foods for Optimum Health*. Rocklin, Calif.: Prima Publishing, 1996.

What I learned from my experience in the development of FITONICS was that *no matter what I ate:*

▶ I needed an **abundance** of fresh fruits, vegetables, and their juices to stay in shape and feel truly energetic.

▶ I needed to eat a wide variety of foods, including **all** the food groups in my diet.

▶ A small amount of animal protein could be a positive element in any eating plan, although my diet remained 90 percent vegetarian.

▶ I needed a natural supplementation progam, including such breakthrough options as enzymes, colloidal minerals, and supernutrients.

▶ My body and psyche required a program that would allow me to enjoy restaurant dining in a nonrestrictive way.

At that point, ten years after the publication of *FIT FOR LIFE,* I was finally clear on how to update that program. My goals were different in the nineties than they had been in the seventies and eighties. Then I had been reaching for health as my overriding goal. Now, I wanted more. I wanted good health, but I also wanted to reverse the aging process, build muscle instead of fat, maintain a youthful figure—and I wanted to do it all with calm and serenity, *quickly* and without being a "slave" in the kitchen or joining the "chain gang" at the gym.

The FITONICS Natural Health Program you will soon be following has given me *all* those results, and you can have them too.

Shattering the Myth
of the Low-Fat Diet

The scientific studies that have led us to the low-fat era in eating have essentially backfired. For many whose concerns I now far better understand, the low-fat message has caused a serious backlash. When studies consistently recommend the reduction of fat, too many of the traditional foods suddenly seem off limits. And the American Dietetic Association reports that the number-one excuse for not eating well is the fear of having to give up a favorite food. The bottom line is that many are unwilling to embrace such radical change in their diets. In fact, the portion of the population motivated to eat a healthful balance of foods has actually slipped by 9 percent since 1991.[2]

Jane Hurley, of the Center for Science in the Public Interest, tells us, "The fast food industry is feeding America's fat tooth." A Triple Decker Pizza at Pizza Hut has more fat oozing out between its layers than a stick and a half of butter. Nearly 25 percent of the $97 billion Americans spent on fast food in 1995 went to the larger, more fattening portions.[3] And when you try to make amends by buying low-fat substitutes, you are receiving just the opposite of what you expect: an unconscionable dose of fattening sugar as a cheap substitute for the fat.

This is one of the main reasons the population is now heavier than when the low-fat trend started ten years ago. You can assess the fallout of low-fat diets when you realize that today the average person eats 10 percent fewer calories than a hundred years ago—a period of time in which the prevalence of obesity has doubled.[4]

Since *FIT FOR LIFE* was published in 1985, our national dietary guidelines, the Four Food Groups, have been replaced by the Eating Right Pyramid, but it is clear that for the 60 million

---

[2]*Self*, January 1996, p. 65.
[3]Bruce Horowitz. "Portion Sizes and Fat Content Out of Control." *USA Today*, February 20, 1996, pp. 1–2.
[4]Kelly Brownell. *Newsweek*, December 5, 1995, p. 60.

obese people in this country these latest government recommendations are not working.

In my opinion, the most important reason for this is the emphasis the Pyramid places on grains as the foundation of our diets, rather than on fruits and vegetables. After over two decades in the diet and health "trenches," I have witnessed repeatedly that unless you are eating *more* fruits and vegetables than any other food, you are probably going to suffer from an excess of fat on your body. There are several other important reasons for why the Pyramid is failing:

▶ Many of the more recent dietary programs published have gone beyond what the Pyramid mandates, lowering fat to 10 percent, making healthful eating seem overly deprivational, or overemphasizing the importance of protein in the diet. These extreme regimens create confusion in the public mind and illness in the body.

▶ You are now supposed to be eating a larger proportion of grains than anything else, and it is recommended that they be *whole* grains. But where do you find those in your supermarket? Certainly not in any great abundance in the bread, cereal, pasta, or rice aisles!

▶ You are supposed to have a minimum of five servings a day of fruits and vegetables. Yet today vegetable consumption is lower than it was a decade ago.[5] Clearly, most Americans still don't understand the many delicious ways to increase the amount of fruits and vegetables in the daily diet.

▶ The Pyramid tells us to use meats, chicken, fish, and dairy as condiments. A population raised to enjoy tubs of fried chicken, racks of ribs, and the sixteen-ounce steak is obviously grappling with how to implement that mandate.

▶ And, finally, fats and sugars, appearing at the very peak of the Pyramid, are to be eaten only sparingly. In my opinion, since so many are reaching for sugary or fatty snacks to assuage hunger caused by nutrient deficiencies, there is no chance we

---

[5]Bernice Kanner: *Parade*, November 12, 1995, p. 4.

will lower our fat and sugar intake in this country until all the other recommendations are being followed in a satisfying way.

Finally, a Solution

The problem is clear: *Too many conflicting dietary guidelines have Americans confused and dissatisfied with the way they are eating.* Understandably, we're all rebelling. Over the years I have seen firsthand how hard it is to last for any length of time on a program that recommends meals that aren't familiar or a shopping list of ingredients that is barely recognizable. After fourteen years of continuous research, I have reached the conclusion that a broad diet—pulling nutrients from a wide range of *wholesome and familiar foods*, including proteins, fats, carbohydrates, and simple sugars—will go farthest to raise the level of health in this country. We need a variety of food from a wide range of sources in our diets to expose our bodies to all possible nutrients necessary for good health.

This is the very program I have developed for you in FITONICS, in recipes for weight loss and health that please the American palate and focus on foods that are easy to prepare from basic affordable ingredients. And since supplementation—in the form of vitamins, minerals, and enzymes—is no longer a luxury but a clear necessity in the quest for natural health, you will find recommendations for the finest, most effective supplement choices.

The Exercise Question and the Answer: BODYTONICS

Too much of what we see on today's exercise scene is bringing confusion to the simple art of being naturally active in life. Complex machines and weights, aerobics classes that demand the coordination of a dancer, and increasingly punishing approaches to the gentle art of yoga are all relegating exercise to the realm of the impossible for nearly three quarters of our population. I myself felt I never had enough time to exercise.

In 1992, when I learned the twelve-to-twenty-minute daily BODYTONICS routines that Donald had developed over a lifetime of study of martial arts, dynamic tension, weight lifting, and yoga, I resolved to help Americans return exercise to its rightful place as an easily integrated part of your daily activity. In my experience, BODYTONICS is a breakthrough. It never gets boring, it never burns you out, and it can put you, like me, in the best shape of your life.

The Soul Needs Feeding Too: MINDTONICS

But the shape of our bodies is not our only preoccupation in this present era. There is a thirst among many in our population for genuine spiritual experience, and it has been proven that such experience can vastly improve our health and increase our happiness.

Millions try to meditate. Unfortunately, it is a difficult process, and as many try to find peace, their minds run in frustrating circles of agitation. I used to sit, sometimes for over an hour, with my mind going round and round before it would finally quiet. After meditation, I found myself going right back to the stressful mental tapes and programs that were not serving me. I knew how important meditation was to me, and I was willing to give it maximum effort, but I didn't know how to maintain the occasional peace and inspiration I found in meditation throughout my day.

MINDTONICS and Hypno-Meditation have strengthened my spiritual connection in my daily life and put me in control of what I create in my world. My meditations are so deep I return from them renewed and able to make better choices in my day which affect my health, happiness, and well-being. MINDTONICS and Hypno-Meditation will help you achieve your goals of weight loss, better health, and happiness.

Putting the Dream into Practice

In October 1993, Donald and I began to teach FITONICS. On the first day, our group shared with us their struggles with their health, the years they had been wrestling with excess weight, and the problems that came from stress in their jobs and relationships. Clearly, these were people searching for a new formula for healthful living.

Ten weeks later, as the video cameras rolled and I looked out into the shining faces of our enthusiastic new friends, I heard myself exclaiming:

"I can't believe I'm fifty years old! I feel like I'm nineteen years old! And I believe with all my heart that this wonderful, youthful feeling is the result of FITONICS!

"I've done a tremendous amount of research on diet and health for over twenty years. I thought I had put it all together into a lifestyle for myself, but the truth is, it hadn't really been working. Everything I was trying to do was too complicated, too demanding, and too time-consuming. But now that I know about Sensible Supplementations, Power Lunches, and Soothing Suppers, things are falling into place. I have MIND-TONICS and Hypno-Meditation! I have BODYTONICS! Using FITONICS to master the body, mind, and spirit to balance my lifestyle is what really changed me. That's what has made me feel like a teenager again!"

That day, as I spoke enthusiastically about my own experiences, much of my excitement was triggered by the incredible transformation I was seeing mirrored in the faces before me. Men and women alike were literally "makeovers" of their former selves. Their skin was clearer and more radiant, their eyes were brighter. They stood straighter and moved with an energy that indicated they felt "no pain." Many had improved relationships. Some had even moved on to better jobs. They were thinner, trimmer, and more toned; all of them were walking and talking in a way that indicated how much better they felt about themselves.

This Is Your Moment

This is *your* moment. This is *your* chance to lose unwanted weight, increase your energy, and embrace a healthier, more fulfilling way of life. Join Donald and me as you turn the page and take control of how you look, feel, and perform every minute of the day. As you watch the pounds melt away and see a strong, happy, energetic person emerge, you'll know it's the time of your life for . . . FITONICS FOR LIFE!

With heartfelt wishes for your success, I reach out to you with love,

Marilyn H. Diamond

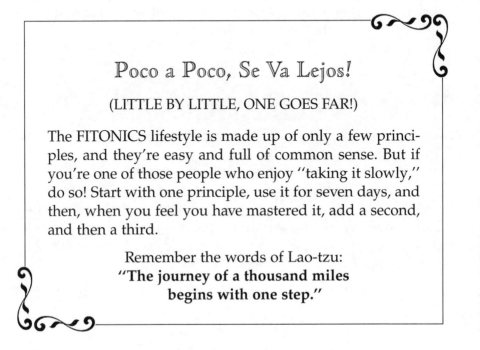

Poco a Poco, Se Va Lejos!

(LITTLE BY LITTLE, ONE GOES FAR!)

The FITONICS lifestyle is made up of only a few principles, and they're easy and full of common sense. But if you're one of those people who enjoy "taking it slowly," do so! Start with one principle, use it for seven days, and then, when you feel you have mastered it, add a second, and then a third.

Remember the words of Lao-tzu:
**"The journey of a thousand miles
begins with one step."**

▼

Introduction

▼

"With FITONICS, I've lost 25 pounds
and I've been able to keep it off.
I think the key to that is its balanced approach.
You have the exercises with BODYTONICS,
the practical way of eating with supplements,
and you also have MINDTONICS,
which help keep you motivated."
—MICHAEL GLASS, ACCOUNTANT
(lost twenty-five pounds in twelve weeks)

Did you pick up this book because you have long dreamed of finding a healthful way of eating? Did you hope to find a plan that would give you a feeling of well-being and satiety while at the same time ensuring weight loss? Have you ever yearned to discover a natural lifestyle that would keep unhealthy fat off your body—perhaps even replace it with some sleek, toned muscle? Did you hope at the same time for a diet that would be pleasurable, without guilt or denial?

That sounds like a fairly tall order, and for most people who have been on the dieting "not-so-merry-go-round" it may also sound like a fairy tale. But you can make this "fairy tale" come true.

A Natural Lifestyle

FITONICS is a natural health lifestyle, designed for all those who are ready to learn how to achieve their diet and health goals naturally and permanently, without deprivation, drugs,

17

or tough regimens. We know this may seem impossible. But we've written this book to show you how *easy* it is—and to tell you, "You *can* do it!"

You have everything you need for success, including time, because the good news about FITONICS is *it doesn't take much time.* You can say good-bye forever to complicated calorie, fat, or carbohydrate counting. You can stop buying meal plans and nutritionally inferior powdered meal substitutes. You can forget the potentially dangerous technique of stomach stapling. There will be no more embarrassing public "weigh-ins." You can be free forever from the promise and hype of a lifetime of weight-loss wonder-drug injections and the inevitable side effects such promises never tell you about.

In short, you can use totally natural, commonsense principles to put your weight and health worries behind you, so you can turn your attention and valuable energy to all the rest and best life has to offer.

Maintain a Healthy Weight Without Dieting

We don't believe you were put here to spend a lifetime struggling with your weight. With FITONICS, eating can become a satisfying, sensible, joyous and rewarding experience—as it was always intended to be—rather than a test of willpower, which, for millions of people, it has become.

To handle your weight and health problems now and forever, FITONICS gives you simple and natural dietary principles that put you in the driver's seat. You use these principles as much as you desire. There are no hard and fast rules. There is no straitjacket. There is no "diet" to blow. You are totally and completely in control. If you digress, just pick up where you left off at your very next meal.

Remember, your body is your vehicle through life. FITONICS is your Owner's Manual. It tells you not only what to do to keep that vehicle in optimal working condition, but also why and how to do it.

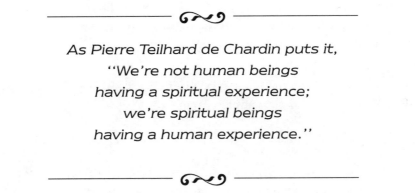

As Pierre Teilhard de Chardin puts it,
"We're not human beings
having a spiritual experience;
we're spiritual beings
having a human experience."

Because we recognize that natural health and spiritual well-being go hand in hand, our goal in developing FITONICS has been your *total* health, achieved naturally.

Benjamin Franklin once said, "An ounce of prevention is worth a pound of cure." As over one-third of our population now embraces alternative and natural approaches to health care, as medicine more and more emphasizes prevention, there is plenty of evidence that prevention through commonsense lifestyle behaviors is the wave of our future. As you follow the FITONICS principles, you will no longer be a pawn to the guessing game when it comes to weight loss and your health.

Our goal for you is *lasting lifestyle changes and results.* And YOU DON'T HAVE TO GET UP FROM THE TABLE HUNGRY! When it comes to the food on your plate, FITONICS is a balanced approach to maximizing your nutrient intake with a wide variety of delicious foods, supported, if you desire, by a program of natural, sensible supplementation. We're excited about helping you return real, nutrient-rich foods to your dinner table.

And when it comes to exercise, it's time to return to *natural* movements in a quick, easy, over-before-you-know-it routine that gives you your healthy look.

We're confident you'll love all the healthful, real-food meals you'll soon be eating. These are the foods that will keep you in shape and give you the energy for productive, happy, and peaceful days. Soon you'll be hearing, as we so often hear, that you look years younger than your age. Imagine how that's going to feel!

Read what Cyndy and Ralph M. from Florida had to say about their success with FITONICS:

> *CYNDY: "I had gotten to the point that I was feeling bad about how old I was. You know, I was thinking, 'This is the way it's got to be.' Then I found FITONICS, and I feel like I'm twenty years old again! I've got that energy. I feel good about myself. I'm ready to go out there and conquer the world again. IT FEELS WONDERFUL! I'm grateful to FITONICS for giving this back to us."*

> *RALPH: "Look at her. She glows now. She looks younger. Her skin has a nicer quality. She looks like she's ready to go."*

> *CYNDY: "I feel like a new person. #1, I'm not hungry. #2, I eat food that I enjoy. #3, best of all, I have lost weight. And he's lost 37 pounds!"*

> *RALPH: "Yep, I'm down from 237 to 200!"*

> *CYNDY: "I feel better about the world, better with our relationship, and even our children are asking, 'What's going on with you two? What's happening?'"*

> *RALPH: "Because they see new parents. I don't know how Marilyn and Don got this idea. I don't care how they got it. All I can say is I'm glad they have and they gave it to me!"*

> *—Cyndy and Ralph M.*
> *(lost fifteen and thirty-seven pounds,*
> *respectively, in nine weeks)*

A Typical FITONICS Day

Here's the innovative FITONICS NATURAL HEALTH FORMULA you'll use to do it:

Each week you'll have the opportunity to focus on main courses of all of the foods you love. You'll have your optional meat days, including optional dairy. There'll be warm-weather juice-and-fruit days for accelerated progress, and cold-weather cleansing days when advances are made with an emphasis on soups and cooked vegetables. You'll have the Funday on Sunday, when you can rest and stretch out—focusing on weight loss even more with fresh, uncooked, natural foods. For those who love vegetarian eating, nonmeat choices are offered throughout.

Here's what a sample day might look like:

▶ To start your morning with energy, help you lose weight, and combat the wilted look and aches and pains that so many attribute to "growing old" but are really the results of nutrient deprivation and too little exercise, you'll begin with the twelve-minute BODYTONICS routine.

▶ Invigorated from these natural movements, you might then have one of our special tonics, a high-energy blend of fruit and juice with the addition of the super-nutrient supplements we recommend. This is a breakfast bursting with natural, wholesome ingredients. Since the majority of our taste buds steer us toward cravings for sweet, we give you "natural sweet" first thing in the morning to handle your cravings throughout the rest of the day.

For those trying to break a sugar addiction, you'll be shocked at how well this works! If you're looking for energy and weight loss, the TONIC is our answer. It staves off hunger for hours and helps stop the unhealthy cravings caused by nutrient deprivation.

▶ For lunch, we encourage you to try the POWER LUNCH,

a high-protein and salad meal to sharpen the mind and stimulate the body, so you won't need an afternoon nap or to reach for caffeinated beverages. You'll have the option of such high-energy super salads as Pasta or Shrimp Salad with Peas, Thai Tofu or Chicken Salad, or Philly Cheese Steak Salad with a bowl of hot soup in winter months.

▶ In the evening we'll be recommending the SOOTHING SUPPER, focusing on complex carbohydrates that will calm you after a busy day. You'll choose from tempting Easy Fajitas or Mashed Potatoes and Gravy Dinner, and you'll love the "soup and sweet" choice. Your meals will be as simple or as elaborate as you desire, and restaurant dining will be a treat you'll still easily enjoy.

What we are going to tell you next is the most fundamental underpinning of Natural Health and the message of FITONICS:

HEALTH CARE IS SELF CARE[1]

The universe is regulated by natural laws.
Your health and proper weight are regulated by
natural health laws.
If you break the laws you will suffer.
In the West, our scientists refer to this idea
as the Law of Cause and Effect.
In the East, this principle is understood as Karma.
For every action, there is an equal and
opposite reaction. . . .
There's no free ride. . . .
Sooner or later, you pay the piper.
If you wish to lose weight and return to health
(if you wish to free up energy for
spiritual evolution),
the way to go about it for the greatest reward
is to respect and apply
the Natural Health principles in this book.

---

[1]"Health Care Is Self Care" is the motto of the American Natural Hygiene Society, which began its pioneering efforts for natural health over sixty years ago.

The Final—and Most Important— Piece of the Puzzle: Enzymes!

FITONICS is designed to bring you the experience of HEALTH CARE IS SELF CARE. That understanding can be a powerful tool for transformation (*when it spurs you to take action*). To make this truth your own, all you need is some basic information. Let's start with the all-important natural law concerning health.

Health is dependent on the quantity of enzymes you have available and the efficient use of these enzymes to activate all the processes in your body that lead to health. And . . . health leads to normalizing your weight! Enzymes are the substances responsible for digestion inside the body. The secret to FITON-ICS is that it adds to your personal enzyme supply. This revolutionary approach to living has never before been presented in the form of a lifestyle program. With FITONICS, you will learn how to use enzyme-rich foods and enzyme supplements to attain good health and the weight loss that naturally follows.

As far back as 1960, in *Today's Health*, published by the *Journal of the American Medical Association,* brilliant medical doctors were saying, "Many researchers believe that the aging process is the result of the slowing down and disorganization of enzyme activity. Might it eventually be possible to restore youthful patterns of activity by supplying those enzymes that are deficient?"

If you are wondering whether we are talking about the Fountain of Youth here, try what we are suggesting and decide for yourself. How will it sound to you when your friends exclaim, "You look so much younger!" As you feel your waistline shrinking, as you tighten your belt and begin buying smaller sizes, you'll be hooked on FITONICS *for Life*! Are you ready to go to the level of excellence in health . . . and in life . . . about which you have often dreamed?

Putting It All Together

If your current lifestyle has made you a master at weight gain, it's time to face the facts: You've also mastered increased risk. Degenerative diseases are at your heels. We hope the latest medical claim that excess weight can be blamed on genetics doesn't end up fostering a national "cop-out." Medicine began blaming all our ills on "germs" at the turn of this century, when the pharmaceutical industry was being born, and we began to hear that profitable "wonder drugs" could fight the diseases we should have been taught to prevent.

Half a century later, the blame shifted from germs to "viruses." Now we're told that the overuse and misuse of antibiotics has caused mutant microbial strains that are literally "immune" to all the drugs we've been taking. The bottom line is that even traditional medical institutions now realize that "fighting" rather than preventing disease isn't lowering disease statistics.

The current trend today is toward "bio-genetics"— the costly new search for faulty genes to explain our illness. While that complicated approach prevails, with decades of research and billions of dollars of funding ahead of it and no practical outcome in sight, aren't you ready for simple solutions TODAY?

In his book *The McDougall Plan*, Dr. John McDougall points out that people from many cultures throughout the world are slender and relatively free from the crippling degenerative diseases that infect America. Dr. McDougall explains that when healthy Chinese of normal weight come to America, they get fat and sick as soon as they imitate our eating habits. Sounds like the problem is an "overloaded plate" gene! Let's not jump too quickly on the "fat gene" theory. Let's use our common sense.

As national health care becomes more costly and elusive, and disorders of the digestive tract account for more hospital admissions than any other group of causes, why not take this opportunity to embrace your power to prevent the cost, pain, and strain of illness and excess weight? In 1977, this statement by the Secretary of Health, Education, and Welfare, published in the *Surgeon General's Report*, set the tone for the conditions of our present era: "You, the individual, can do more for your own health and well-being than any doctor, any hospital, any drug, and exotic medical device."

This, in our opinion, is the most relevant prescription for natural health as we move toward the new millennium.

As you embrace FITONICS, you will realize that it is, in truth, your own personal health care program. AND AS YOU GAIN HEALTH, YOU LOSE WEIGHT naturally. As you now begin your own FITONICS adventure, we welcome you to the first day of the rest of your healthier, happier life.

PART ONE

A NUTRITIONAL BREAKTHROUGH

1

▼

Diets Still Don't Work

▼

"One of the reasons the program works
is because you don't feel you're deprived all the time.
You're not always craving something
you think you can never have again.
Which is why diets don't work.
It's why FITONICS does work!"
—PATTI E., *ACTRESS*

Every year an estimated 80 million Americans go on diets. No matter how much weight they lose, 95 percent of them gain it all back.[1] If you are one of them, our hearts are with you, and our intention with FITONICS is to free you **forever** from that traumatic human experience.

The causes of failure are the common motivations behind dieting: fear, frustration, and anger. You're afraid you're going to have a heart attack. You detest the way your clothes look on you. You blame every setback in your life on your excess weight. You make the fat on your body the demon. You are full of self-hate because of it and you vow to starve yourself. You'll never eat anything fattening again. YOU'RE GOING ON A DIET!

Before long, to mask your hunger, you're reaching for cigarettes and living on diet sodas. You've traded the joy of sitting down to a real meal for junky diet bars and nonnutritious shakes. At the supermarket, you allow yourself to buy only

---

[1]Philip Elmer-Dewitt. "Fat Times." *Time*, January 1995.

low-fat this and nonfat that, foods that promise you'll be slim "fast"; but you find yourself overeating because you just don't feel satisfied. You're stuffing yourself with dry bagels and plain pasta, while you're continuously craving ice cream, pizza, peanut butter and jelly sandwiches, and all the other "fattening" foods your body has for years been habituated to consume. You're less and less enthusiastic, low on energy, and irritable, but you persevere—because you **have** somehow lost four pounds.

For the first time in six months, you go to the gym you joined on your birthday. You're overheated, flushed, sweating, and humiliated. You know you've got a lo-o-o-ng way to go.

After three or four weeks, you snap one night. You go out to the all-night convenience store "to buy a newspaper" and you find yourself gobbling cookies or Danish and buying two quarts of extra-rich ice cream that you know you're about to consume. The next day, you order the double cheeseburger, large french fries, and the turnover; and for dinner, you dig into a tub of fried chicken, mashed potatoes, and biscuits.

Now it's over. In two weeks you're five pounds heavier than when you started. You're afraid to step on a scale. You avoid mirrors and cancel your membership at the health club. You're embarrassed to see your friends. You're angry at yourself, wishing THEY had *never* invented food. You're convinced you'll never succeed at losing weight. YOUR MIND IS LITERALLY BEATING YOU UP!

Fear, embarrassment and anger are not health-promoting emotions. They come from psychological and physical stress and they generate more of the same. Ironically, stress is an appetite stimulator. We reach for food in an attempt to soothe our nerves. Depriving ourselves of food only causes more stress. We're in that vicious cycle: a few pounds off, a few more on. The problem becomes more deep-seated each time a diet fails. Self-esteem drops. You feel like a moral failure. You know everyone is thinking:

"She looked so good for a while, but she blew it again."

"He sure doesn't seem to have the inner strength to stick to it. . . . Doesn't he care about his appearance?"

You *do* care, and your desperation is silently mounting. You read in a magazine that you may have a "genetic problem," and you lunge for that explanation. Even though your inner voice is telling you, "No, I don't."

"One quarter of the deaths in the Nurses' Health Study were attributable to obesity. The latest results from the study of 115,000 nurses showed that a moderately to severely overweight woman (such as a 5'5" woman who weighs more than 175 lbs.) was more than twice as likely to die prematurely as a thin woman."
—*Self*, January 1996

In 1985, 25 percent of all Americans were overweight. Today that figure has climbed to 33 percent.[2] Have our genes somehow mysteriously transformed in one decade? Of course not. How is it, then, that what was a one-in-four statistic for obesity only ten years ago is now one in three?

Why We Are Heavier Than Ever

Here are two simple explanations:

1. As a population, we haven't yet learned to defend ourselves against the **real** demons. The sad truth is, most of us can't even recognize real food any longer. We have allowed ourselves to be persuaded that packages of devitalized, fractionated, and synthetic "substances" we're eating in place of real food have nothing to do with our poor health and obesity statistics.

   In this area, we need a commonsense wake-up call. If the ingredients of what you are eating don't occur naturally . . .

---

[2]Dr. C. Everett Koop. "America's Health at Risk: A Call to Action." *Time*, May 1995.

IT'S NOT FOOD! That means that if what you are eating is described by a mile-long list of words you can't pronounce, you're not eating **food!** If it doesn't grow out of the ground or on a tree; if it doesn't come from natural sources, from the fields, meadows, or oceans; if it is clear that it is a laboratory creation—YOU'RE NOT EATING FOOD!

Beware of wolves in sheep's clothing. When something you're eating contains more chemicals and additives than it does real food sources, you're being had. We're the only country in the world with supermarkets full of fake foods and a population that lives primarily on an artificial diet, and we're the ones with the weight problems. We've been duped into believing that if we eat low-fat "cardboard" versions of cake, nonfat "plastic" versions of ice cream, and bags of chips loaded with "fake fat," we're actually doing something good for ourselves.

By the way, of 23,000 adults surveyed in sixteen states, only 20 percent were eating five or more servings of fruits and vegetables a day.[3] Vegetable consumption is actually *dropping*. Ten years ago, 53 percent of meals served at home came with a vegetable side dish; today, only 44 percent do.[4]

2. Most of our population has not yet learned how to replace destructive eating habits with constructive ones. The problem is confounded by all the contradictory and erroneous information about what exactly constitutes "healthy eating habits." You're told to count calories, count fat grams, count carbohydrates, substitute artificial foods, increase your protein, eliminate entire food groups, weigh your food, control your portions—and *none of this can lead to natural health and permanent weight loss.*

For years, we have watched overweight consumers in the supermarkets loading their shopping carts with diet sodas

---

[3]*Environmental Nutrition*, November 1995, p. 4.
[4]Bernice Kanner. *Parade*, November 12, 1995, p. 4.

and iced teas, diet frozen food dinners, and diet snacks. If you're doing this, you're making changes, but not the *right* ones.

The point is: You can count calories, you can watch fat grams, you can waste your money on diet pills, but until you understand exactly which foods build health in your body and which build *ill-health,* what you are doing for your health is the same as trying to repair your car with duct tape.

Please, forget about "diet foods," "diet pills," and overworking yourself at the gym—and please, don't consider the Natural Health lifestyle that unfolds on the pages that follow a diet. It's a tried and proven, normal, sensible way to live to build health and lose weight. One of the most gratifying experiences we had during the FITONICS test was working with women who had been struggling for years to lose weight they gained during pregnancy. They'd tried one diet after another, but it wasn't until they embraced the lifelong guidelines of FITONICS that those ten to twenty pounds were history!

"The FDA will allow any pharmaceutical company that wants to to claim a new drug is 'safe' (there is no prescription drug sold that is 100% safe) and results in an absolute weight-loss of 5% total body weight.

"My aunt Sylvia is 5'5" and weighs 120 lbs. If she visits her physician to ask for a prescription for a new weight-loss drug (office visit: $50) and then takes the drug for one year (about $600), she has spent $650 to lose 6 pounds. Someone is getting rich and it's not my Aunt Sylvia. . . .

"Why would the FDA want to approve the sale of a drug, complete with side effects, to trusting Americans desperate to shed excess body weight?"

—Robert Haas, Ph.D., "Eat to Win," *Muscular Development,* February 1996

Diets Are Temporary Solutions and Temporary Solutions Bring Only Temporary Results

You can use this lifestyle for two weeks if you choose, and you'll be lighter and fit better into your clothes as a result. But you'll also have a new glow in your skin, a shine in your eyes, a feeling of returning health and vitality, that you won't want to lose.

You get these benefits only from following the path to natural health. You can try to use what you find in this book as a diet, but once you've experienced the many benefits it brings in addition to weight loss, you'll want it to be as much a part of your life as love, friendship, romance, happiness, wealth, success, and all the other positive human experiences you'd never think to limit to two-week doses. You'll want FITONICS for Life!

What About You?

In 1994, two Harvard researchers, Drs. Per Bjorntorp and Theodore Vanltallie, analyzed the impact of worldwide obesity on five diseases: cardiovascular, diabetes, hypertension, osteoarthritis, and gallbladder disease, and conservatively estimated the cost to be $45.8 billion annually. That's a financial drain the world cannot afford.

Every year 400,000 Americans die prematurely from cigarette smoking. But few people realize that obesity is directly responsible for over 300,000 untimely deaths during the same time period, placing excess body fat second only to smoking as a cause of preventable death.[5]

---

[5]Robert Haas. "Eat to Win." *Muscular Development*, February 1996, p. 40.

Obesity is the root cause of the largest proportion of the degenerative diseases that are wiping out three of four Americans. We are literally killing ourselves as we tuck in our napkins. Our wounds are inflicted with our knives and forks. Excess weight contributes largely to five of the ten leading causes of death in the United States, including heart disease, high blood pressure, stroke, diabetes, and some cancers. Clearly, excess pounds are no longer just a matter of vanity. They're a very real threat to life. As you turn the page, you are taking your first step toward the **only** solution your common sense will embrace. You are entering the world we lost only recently, the world that has been the domain of our species since the beginning of time. You are returning to your original state of . . .

2

▼

Natural Health

▼

". . . it appears to me necessary
to every physician to be skilled in nature,
and to strive to know,
if he would wish to perform his duties,
what a man is in relation to the articles
of food and drink, and to his other occupations,
and what are the effects of each of them to every one,
Whoever does not know what effect
these things produce upon a man
cannot know the consequences
which result from them.
Whoever pays no attention to these things,
or paying attention, does not comprehend them,
how can he understand the diseases which befall a man?
For, by every one of these things
a man is affected and charged this way and that,
and the whole of his life is subjected to them,
whether in health, convalescence, or disease.
Nothing else, then, can be
more important than these things."
—HIPPOCRATES

It's the only state of being that absolutely *guarantees* you will not have a weight problem. Excess weight is not your *natural* condition. Excess weight is *unnatural*. If you lived in Nature, there would be absolutely no way you could drag excess weight, and the diseases it creates, around with you. That's what "survival of the fittest" is all about. Have you ever seen an overweight giraffe? A plump coyote? Their only potential for excess weight is when they're living *unnaturally* in captivity.

You Come from Strong Stock

To survive in Nature, you must be able to aggressively pull your own weight. If you are saddled with more than you can comfortably handle, there is no possibility of meeting Nature's challenges.

Think about it. You're out in the wild, without food or shelter. Civilization, as you know it, doesn't exist. There are no Days Inns or 7-Elevens, no Stage Delicatessens or Burger Kings, no cellular phones, freeways, minivans, or subways. It's up to you to take care of all your needs from what Nature provides.

If you can't walk for miles, climb hills and mountains, ford icy streams, run from predators, forage and hunt, build your shelter, and clothe yourself, can you survive? Probably not! However, the only reason you're here today is because your ancestors *could*. You carry their genes within you.

Your biological encoding, which is another way of saying "the natural state of your species," is not one of disease or overweight. Your biological encoding is for survival, and do you think for one minute, as part of your natural survival mechanism, that your body is lacking the natural ability to shed excess weight? All that stands in its way is your lack of knowledge and application of the principles of Natural Health.

The Natural Health Pioneers

In a culture that has elevated disease to the most profitable business on earth, the torch for Natural Health has been carried by health pioneers who lived robustly into their nineties or more without the problems of excess weight, cancer, diabetes, hypertension, strokes, or heart attacks. Many of these pioneers, men and women alike, were naturopathic physicians and chiropractors, and some of the greatest contributions came from medical doctors.

In most cases, these pioneers devoted their entire adult lives—as we have done—to gathering the kernels of wisdom and truth about natural living to pass on to future generations. At the root of all their teaching is a basic principle, which is the very foundation of the Natural Health philosophy.

Only Nature Heals

Now, what does that mean in practical terms? Your body has the power and intelligence to grow, on its own, from a tiny ovum to a full-sized adult. It has the innate ability, as well, to keep itself perfectly healthy and at a normal weight. And, if you don't push it too far into disease, it has the innate ability to heal, rejuvenate, and repair itself. All you need to do is make your best efforts, as often as possible, to supply it with the elements Nature provides for your body's survival. What are those elements? Fresh air, pure water, wholesome and fresh natural foods, regular exercise, adequate rest and sleep, peaceful and supportive surroundings, and a higher spiritual connection. All of these elements are far easier, more likely pain free, and far less expensive to attain than the traumatically invasive treatments they will help you prevent.

In other words, whatever your health goals may be, especially if one is weight loss, the secret to reaching them is to take a new, nurturing, caretaking role in your relationship with your body.

Natural Health Equals Normal Weight

If it's weight loss you are seeking, become naturally healthier and your weight problem will be handled by the natural forces for health within you.

⟨⟨~⟩⟩

*The goal, therefore, is not just
the "sporting" of a fashionably
thin body.
The goal is a
strong, well-nourished body—
a healthful, natural weight.*

⟨⟨~⟩⟩

This basic understanding may not presently be at the core of your thinking about health because you are living in a society that has pursued obsessive skinniness and unnatural measures to attain health for several generations. The focus on drugs and surgery, starvation diets, appetite suppressants, and bingeing and purging shows that we fight the symptoms rather than removing the causes.

Society programs you to ignore the obvious problem—the distance you have put between yourself and the natural living habits that are the biological heritage of your species. Rather than preventing excess weight and disease, you've pursued them by deliberately or unknowingly embracing the lifestyle that guarantees them.

Along the way, more programming has taught you to approve of "thin at any cost" and to disregard

"Cardiovascular disease is America's leading killer of both men and women, causing over 40 percent of all deaths. The cause of heart attacks and arteriosclerosis is a twentieth-century disease brought about by modern lifestyles and diet changes to fat-rich, animal-derived foods. Because arteriosclerosis is diet-related, it affects all ages. In 1993, a study of trauma victims who died at the age of 15 showed that all had fatty streaks in their arteries. Of those who died at an average age of 26, nearly 80 percent had evidence of heart blockage."

—Otis-Clapp Pharmaceuticals brochure, P.O. Box 9160, Canton, Mass. 02021

the most conspicuous signs of true health: strength; muscle tone; bright, clear eyes; radiant skin; spontaneous smiles; and the peaceful, focused, optimistic mental state that is the natural human condition in good times and bad. If this state is possible for some, it is certainly possible for you.

Every day that you actively pursue your natural state of health, you are moving toward the fullest expression of your evolutionary potential in body, mind, and spirit. When you move away from the healthy self, you reap the disease and depression so many are experiencing.

Natural Health:
A Celebration of Life

Exactly what is Natural Health? Before you can wholeheartedly embrace it, you have to understand it. *Natural Health is the perfect balance of body, mind, and spirit.* It includes a normalized weight, boundless energy, and a clear and happy mind. Therefore, if you are overweight and you begin to follow the principles of Natural Health, weight loss is one of the assured side effects. A dramatic increase in vitality and well-being are inevitable benefits.

When you are naturally healthy, you are able to find a peaceful place within yourself in the most tumultuous surroundings, a sense of connection to everyone you meet. Natural Health is the tendency to seek the good in every situation and every human being and to focus on the harmonious and constructive. It's a spiritual paradigm for life that balances our Western emphasis on the material. It's a state of lovingness that is unconditional. It's the ability to truly enjoy every aspect of human existence to the fullest, a *joie de vivre* that can't be denied.

Why does healthy make you happy? Because you feel so clean, so light, so full of energy. You can't help but bring this energy to every situation you encounter. If your body is not at its highest level of energy and nourishment, how can you hold the highest thoughts, aspirations, and visions? You can't when your body, *your temple*, is dragging you down.

There's so much ill health in this country, so much *imbalance* and negativity, and so much of a tendency to promote them that there's a good chance you've never even had the opportunity to be face-to-face with Natural Health. When you are with someone who is naturally healthy, you may sense within you an unusual attraction. You want to plug into the energy, enthusiastic clarity of purpose, and the radiance you are detecting. Deep inside, you know you are witnessing your own true nature in another human being.

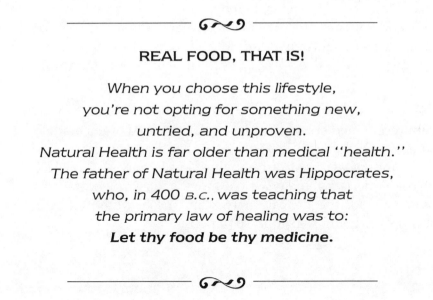

REAL FOOD, THAT IS!

When you choose this lifestyle,
you're not opting for something new,
untried, and unproven.
Natural Health is far older than medical "health."
The father of Natural Health was Hippocrates,
who, in 400 B.C., was teaching that
the primary law of healing was to:
Let thy food be thy medicine.

A New Body Every Year

What Hippocrates was saying was: "Your body will heal and repair, *if* it is given the proper nourishment. Proper nourishment obviously means only what can contribute to the building of cells that number, according to Dr. Deepak Chopra, around

50 trillion strong.[1] These cells are constantly breaking down, constantly giving you the opportunity to build new ones.

Chopra relates: "Ninety-eight percent of the atoms in your body were not there a year ago. The skeleton that seems so solid was not there three months ago. The skin is new every month. You have a new stomach lining every four days."[2]

Dr. Michael Colgan writes, "Every year over 97 percent of your body is completely replaced, even the structure of the DNA of your genes, reconstructed entirely from the nutrients you eat."[3]

Do you realize what an opportunity this is? If you give your body the elements of Natural Health every day—pure whole-food sources of proteins, carbohydrates, fats, vitamins, minerals, and enzymes; plenty of clean water; fresh air (oxygen); regular exercise and meditation; and adequate relaxation and sleep—you will live a long, disease-free life full of youthful vim and vigor.

The word *natural* is the opposite of the word *artificial*. In this unprecedented era of artificial and engineered foods made from unnatural, chemical ingredients, every time you reach for this "chemical feast" you are moving away from Natural Health. Most Americans today drink more soda than water. Think about it. All the delicate nerves and tissues the bloodstream bathes are being soaked in soda pop!

Physical Activity Is Natural

The human body, from its beginnings, has been accustomed to natural exercise in the form of hunting, gathering, and the strenuous work required before the "push-button" era of high tech-

---

[1]Deepak Chopra. *Quantum Healing*. New York: Bantam Books, 1989, p. 3.
[2]Ibid., p. 48.
[3]Michael Colgan. *The New Nutrition*. Encinitas: C.I. Publications, 1994, p. 78.

nology. Sadly, though, only a tiny portion of our population is involved in the kind of exertion that pumps fresh air into the lungs.

The largest number of Americans are stagnating in the pollution of their own oxygen-poor blood. For the first time in human history, human beings are a sedentary species! As well, we habitually rob our bodies of the sleep that is a key element to our survival. Rather than sleeping the natural hours from sundown to sunrise, we prolong the day well into the night with enervating television in the name of relaxation. Those precious hours of sleep so many are willing to compromise are the "prime time" your body has for building all the new cells we are talking about.

Given these unfortunate cultural habits, what kind of new cells do you think you are building? Let's say that the building of healthy new cells is a profession for which you are being paid. At your present level of performance, how long do you think you'd keep your job? Hippocrates admonished us that our food should be our remedy. What does that tell you about the present approach to health in this country? Perhaps you'll agree that it's anything but natural.

Unnatural living habits lead us to the surgeon's knife. They propel us in the direction of pharmaceutical drugs and a litany of side effects requiring more drugs.

You may ask, "What choice do I have? I live in New York (or Los Angeles). What could be more unnatural than that?"

Right! Precisely! We've written this book for you! You need to embrace as much natural living in as many areas of your life as you can, in order to tip the scale in your favor. This means you need regular natural exercise—such as BODYTONICS— which allow for the toning of all your muscles. You need natural food, fresh fruits and vegetables, pure water, whole grains, lean proteins, and legumes. You need peaceful moments for recharging your body, mind, and spirit, and you owe it to yourself to find adequate time for sleep.

In other words, your unnatural surroundings are a wake-up call to give yourself as much *natural support* as you can to offset the disadvantages of your environment. We know this is true because we speak from experience. Both of us reached out for Natural Health when the environments of our lives were the most demanding—and, in many ways, unnatural and un-healthy.

Natural Health Has a History

Natural Health was strong in our country in the 1800s. Back then, our democratic roots supported freedom of choice in health care and physicians of many fields—naturopathy and homeopathy, herbologists, and hygienists—all enjoyed popu-larity among the people. These were the healing professions that women, in particular, practiced, and their clienteles were large and enthusiastic.

In 1848, a small group of upper-class white male doctors—who called themselves "regular" doctors to set themselves apart from other physicians, and who primarily catered to the wealthy—incorporated an organization known as the American Medical Association. However, the official-sounding title belied the lack of interest everyday Americans showed for the caustic drugs, bleedings, and other debilitating methods of treatment that were their specialty in that era.

The early AMA's proclaimed goal and strategy was to squash all competition and monopolize the market. The people fought back, waging a Popular Health Revolution, rallying for freedom of choice with the battle cry for Natural Health.

▶ In the mid-1800s, with the population barely reaching 17 million, *3 million men and women* (accounting for 17.6 percent of the population!) were subscribing to the Thomsonian herbal formulas and publications called *Family Rights*, developed by Samuel Thomson and a female herbologist.[4]

---

[4]Jeanne Achterberg. *Woman As Healer*. Boston: Shambala, 1990, p. 141.

▶ There were 2,500 homeopathic physicians—with hundreds of thousands of followers, most of whom were women—who had their own "domestic kits" containing numbered vials for diagnosis and treatment.[5]

▶ Hydrotherapy (the use of water fasts, mineral baths, and colonics), developed by Mary Grove Nichols, a protégé of Sylvester Graham (of graham cracker fame), was taught to mothers in an effort to raise the standard of health and hygiene.

Contrary to popular medical "mythology," it is to those efforts that we can look for the lessening of infectious disease at the turn of the century, and not to the drugs and treatments the AMA was advocating.

Many "regular" medical doctors, as standard-bearers for AMA policy, sanctioned alcohol consumption and tobacco usage and ridiculed

> By December 31, 1995, of the 720,325 licensed physicians in this country, only 296,361 belonged to the AMA.

the advice of Natural Health proponents for fresh air, frequent bathing, and personal hygiene. They warned an unknowing public about the "dangers" of fresh fruits and vegetables, and ridiculed the emphasis Natural Health physicians placed on fresh wholesome diets, exercise, pure air, nonbinding clothing, and abstention from alcohol and cigarettes.

But "regular" doctors did not have the ear of many of our leading citizens. Among those who encouraged the natural prevention rather than the medical treatment of disease were Mark Twain, John Harvey Kellogg (the cereal king), Mary Baker Eddy (the founder of the Christian Science Church), Ellen White (prophetess of the Seventh-Day Adventist Church), Henry Ford, and Dr. Oliver Wendell Holmes. Holmes once declared that if all the doctors' drugs were thrown into the sea, it would be so much better for humankind and so much worse for the fish.

---

[5]Ibid., p. 142.

Hey! We Thought This Was a Democracy!

So, although many of our American forefathers and foremothers were enthusiastic practitioners of Natural Health, early in the twentieth century freedom of choice in health care eluded our population. A burgeoning pharmaceutical industry supporting the ambitious and monopolistic AMA used legislative clout to force all "drugless" competition out of business and underground.

The reason we are struggling with excess weight, disease and the idea of prevention today, and the explanation for why there is no meaningful government support for precious little but drugs and other medical treatments, can be directly traced to the official closing of all schools of Natural Health and to the revocation of licensing for all but medical doctors.

As a result of the political muscle of an "old boy" network between politicians and the medical/pharmaceutical industry, a series of documented monopolistic practices that led to aggressive and hostile campaigns literally wiped out the voice of Natural Health. Consequently, we lost the knowledge of how to prevent obesity and maintain our normal weight.

Until the 1980s, well-meaning but politically brainwashed medical doctors would push irrational dieting as a solution for weight loss. They would undervalue exercise. At the same time, surgery and pharmaceuticals were the only options in health care. Medical doctors would tell their suffering patients that there was no relationship between disease and diet, or any other lifestyle choice.

While the AMA-driven government health policy created the myth that yet one more breakthrough or wonder drug would bail us out of our disease predicament (if we'd only spend a few billion dollars more on "health" care), Natural Health pioneers quietly kept the *home fires of prevention* burning.

They've fought against the medical establishment's resistance to policies of prevention right up to the present moment.

The AMA vs. Chiropractic

Chiropractic treatment as a means to keep energy flowing in the body directly contributes to prevention of disease and is an important player in the field of Natural Health. In 1986, in *Wilke v. AMA*, the American Medical Association was convicted in federal court of being *the largest professional violator of the Sherman antitrust laws* after a three-decade-long campaign to discredit and undermine its most threatening competitor, the field of chiropractic. A permanent injunction order against the American Medical Association by Federal Court Judge Susan Getzendammer was published in the prestigious *Journal of the American Medical Association* in January 1988.

Further rulings on the case against the AMA appeared in the September, May, and January 1988 issues. The three chiropractors who brought that suit against the monolithic AMA and its bevy of defense attorneys and $6 million legal budget specifically requested no damages, so that financial gain could never be interpreted as the reason for the suit. The only stipulation asked by chiropractic was that the ruling against AMA monopolistic policies be published in the AMA's own journal.

The AMA vs. Supplementation

Every decade since the 1960s, consumers have been forced to fight against AMA-supported legislation to remove all nutritional supplements from the shelves and give them over to medical doctors exclusively as profit-making, prescriptive medicines. That would mean that you could not buy a bottle of vitamin C without a visit to the doctor and a doctor's prescription! Insult to Injury! Less than 12 percent of medical schools require courses in nutrition and other factors in disease prevention, yet you would be relying on those with that limited background for guidance on nutrient intake for health.

Chiropractors study nutrition extensively. Naturopaths and doctors of *ayurveda* and Oriental medicine study nutrition. Why then put nutritional supplements exclusively under the jurisdiction of the surgical and pharmaceutical experts? Our food is already devitalized, and the nutritional supplements we need to stay healthy are under threat of being taken out of easy access! Why would this be happening? Who's really behind it? Who has the most to gain from it? Perhaps the usage of supplements by over 100 million people is posing some direct competition to the industry.

Some of you might have the opinion that people don't know how to take vitamins and could be unknowingly poisoning themselves, and that's why a medical doctor needs to be in charge. Dr. Michael Colgan, a leading specialist in nutritional supplementation, mounts a powerful argument against this idea:

"The strongest evidence for the safety of nutrient supplements is found in the annual reports of the Poison Control Centers. For the years 1985–1990, poison emergencies with medical drugs killed 2,251 people. Simple analgesics, such as aspirin, killed 640 people.

"I say emergencies because the number of deaths caused each year by 'normal' use of drugs is enormous. In hearings before Representative Elton Gallegly on February 18, 1994, Mitchell Zeller of the FDA coolly announced that the number of deaths in America from 'normal' use of prescription drugs is an estimated 150,000 per year. That is an obscene 900,000 deaths between 1985 and 1990. Publicly, the FDA keeps very quiet about these figures, because they approved the prescription drugs' use in the first place.

"In the same period, nutrient supplements now used by more than 100 million Americans every day killed one person—by overdose of niacin. Used in any sensible amounts, vitamins and minerals are about as toxic as apple pie."[6]

Hospitals Could Serve Us Better

Natural Health practitioners specializing in prevention and the noninvasive alleviation of symptoms are denied full hospital privileges and their services are not covered by health insurance in most regions of this country. Those with medical insurance coverage who wish to seek natural treatments for prevention are frequently denied insurance coverage.

Chiropractic, naturopathy, homeopathy, medical hypnotherapy, acupuncture, and massage therapy—all effective measures for the prevention and treatment of certain illnesses and the lessening of painful symptoms—are not yet integrated into hospital protocol. Millions of suffering hospital patients would rest easier and heal faster if such measures were given their due place in treatment.

> "Over one million patients are injured in hospitals each year and approximately 180,000 die annually as a result of these injuries."[7]

Finally, as an example of how far we strayed from the principles of Natural Health, we need only to look at birthing practices in this country. The American College of Obstetricians and Gynecologists officially opposes midwifery. Yet, our country shows poorly in infant and maternal mortality rates as compared to Europe, where midwives practice more readily.

Jeanne Achterberg writes: ". . . In Holland, where over one-third of the births are attended by midwives, the mortality rates are among the lowest in the world. (The actual mortality rates

---

[6]Colgan. *The New Nutrition*, pp. 107–108.
[7]Ibid., pp. 107–108.

in the United States have improved slightly over the decade; however, the relative position among industrialized countries is still close to the last, behind the European countries, Canada and Hong Kong.)"[8]

While midwives in our country are thwarted in their attempts to obtain malpractice insurance, "to date, only 6 percent of nurse midwives have been sued, whereas 66.9 percent of obstetricians have been sued at least once, according to the American College of Obstetricians and Gynecologists."[9]

Don't Blame the Doctors

This is not to belittle the dedicated individual practitioners, doctors, nurses, paramedics, and all the supporting medical staff who are on call to handle the thousands of medical emergencies that take place every hour of every day. If you or a loved one are in an accident, who will be there day or night to save you? The medical doctors in this country are some of the finest in the world. The political maneuverings of the system behind them is what demands our scrutiny. And our own efforts are demanded as well. Our doctors are under pressure and our system is overloaded because of poor lifestyle choices. With simple principles of Natural Health, you can now do your part.

As Natural Health modalities struggle to overcome the obstacles raised against their attempts to bring their services to the public, the resulting belief among millions of Americans is that many of these services are somehow inferior to *any* form of medical treatment. This is not the fault of individual medical doctors but rather of the political and profit-driven system that controls them.

---

[8]Achterberg. *Woman As Healer*, p. 183.
[9]Ibid., p. 182.

In lecturing about the AMA policy of repression of natural forms of therapy and prevention, a noted naturopath, Dr. Paul Bragg, always said, "A thousand years hence, the message of Natural Health will be as up-to-date as at this hour. The methods of living based on the laws of Mother Nature are always in order and never become obsolete."

> The *Journal of the American Medical Association* reports that with 4,383 sick days out of the average seventy-six-year life span, Americans can expect to have about twelve unhealthy years.

It's Time for Action

In 1950, American life expectancy ranked seventh in the world—behind Norway, the Netherlands, Sweden, Denmark, New Zealand, and Australia. In 1990, we ranked eighteenth![10] Today we rank twenty-sixth![11] Among the countries ahead of us are Japan (in the number-one position), Switzerland, Spain, Italy, Sweden, the Netherlands, France, Greece, Canada, Norway, Germany, Austria, Belgium, Australia, England/Wales, and Denmark.

At twenty-sixth, we live to the average age of seventy-five, while the Japanese average is seventy-nine. Yet we pay twice as much for health care as the Japanese![12] At the present rate of expenditure, our medical bills will soon equal nearly *20 percent* of our gross national product!

Dr. Roy Walford, the renowned longevity researcher at UCLA, believes that with proper care our bodies are designed to live for at least 120 years. We agree, and wholeheartedly embrace his findings—and we don't think that means being hooked up to a machine at a debilitating dollar price tag until we finally succumb to what is called "Harvard" death. Dr. Wal-

---

[10]Colgan. *The New Nutrition*, pp. 42–44.
[11]Peter Jaret. "When East Feeds West." *Eating Well*, November 1995, p. 34.
[12]Colgan. *The New Nutrition*, pp. 42–44.

ford is not talking about an extended life that 50 percent of our population is now destined for—according to the Centers for Disease Control—a life ending with many years in a nursing home. His is a much happier, healthier scenario entirely.

The principles of Natural Health you will soon be learning offer the opportunities for easy and healthful weight loss and a long, productive, disease-free life. Join the FITONICS Natural Health Revolution! Be among those of us who plan to live our lives with our running shoes on, rather than in hospital slippers. You can start immediately by understanding that the ultimate commodity for your health is . . .

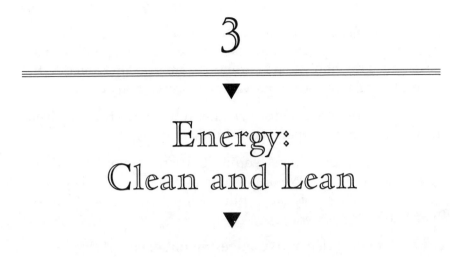

3

▼

Energy: Clean and Lean

▼

Energy is the essence of your life. There is no process in your body that can go on without it. Understanding energy, how to avoid wasting it, and how to consistently build it will make all the difference as to whether you are healthy or sick, slim or overweight, happy or depressed. If your goal is a lean, dynamic body, there is no possibility of success if you are low in energy.

Energy travels through your nerves to activate every cell in your blood, bones, organs, and tissues. If your nerve force is high, then, in all likelihood, you're a healthy, happy camper.

What the old-time chiropractors, some of the early Natural Health pioneers, taught is essentially correct. Picture nerve force as water and the nerves as a garden hose. If the supply of water is low or cut off, what happens to the garden? In the same way, what happens to your organs, which are composed of cells, if they don't receive enough energy in the form of nerve force? Metaphorically, they "wilt."

Life Is Energy

Life flows through your nerves as energy. When your energy is high, you have no problem meeting the world's challenges. You don't suffer from excess weight. You have your health. You are able to do whatever you wish without having to "pass" on opportunity or experience because you're too "pooped" to play. Your strength, vitality, and endurance are directly related to the quantity and free flow of nerve force in your body.

The quality of your life—whether it will be rich with adventure and reward—depends on abundant energy.

▶ Good relationships require it. There cannot be fulfilling sex without energy. Wouldn't your mate be happier if you responded with passionate enthusiasm, instead of "I'm exhausted"?

▶ Parenting demands a huge amount of energy.

▶ Your upward mobility in your profession is completely energy-dependent. (Who, after all, is going to get the best job or a promotion? The person who drags around the office, barely able to make it through the day? Or the one with pep, get-up-and-go, and determination?)

▶ A woman's beauty is the result of abundant nerve force that energizes the cells of her skin, radiates from her eyes, and makes her glow.

▶ A man's muscularity and virility are energy-dependent. Good muscle tone depends upon good nerve force.

Nerve force—ENERGY—
is behind all that is worthwhile
and positive in your life.

Who Rules the World?

If you awaken every morning feeling dull and tired, old and fatigued, with no ambition or excitement for the day, if your future looks hopeless and dark, then you are out of energy. You are one of the 95 percent that Natural Health pioneer Dr. Paul Bragg described when he taught that 5 percent of the people rule the other 95 percent. They are the 5 percent with the most energy!

All stress equals a drain on your energy, and at no time in our history have we exposed ourselves to stress in so many new ways. How often have you heard friends and family members testifying to their lack of energy?

"My nerves are shot!"

"I can't handle any more."

What about you? How often do you say that?

We see little children sitting passively for hours, entranced by television. We see idle teenagers sitting in malls with nothing better to do than smoke. Many of their mothers and fathers, after a draining day's work or a "bear of a week," are crashed in front of television sets at home. The low energy within all of them is apparent. They're part of the 95 percent.

Activity Builds Energy

We are the most sedentary population in any time in history. Our national average for television is six hours per day. Almost *half* of the waking hours of every day! That's an *average*, mind you. While you may be watching less, equal numbers are watching even more than six hours! Add to that the additional hours on-line and on the phone.

Artificial Foods Drain Energy

Furthermore, we fill our bodies with overly processed and denatured foods. These are lacking in the nutrients our cells need to be healthy. In other words, these foods lack ENERGY. They're not going to give you any bang for your buck. If you're wondering which foods we're talking about, here's a very partial list:

Diet soda	Diet iced tea
White bread	White sugar
Donuts	Candy bars
Pretzels	Potato chips
Cotton candy	Jell-O
Sugary cereals	Fried foods

It is stressful for our cells to be fed but still starved of nutrients. We are living at a time in human evolution when we are subjecting our bodies to more unnatural food than ever before. This is creating massive stress in epidemic proportions—*and a paralyzing lack of energy.*

The more stress to your body, the less energy you will have. If you are trying to lose weight or improve your health, there is no possibility for success if you are low on energy.

Weight Loss Requires Energy

It takes energy to eliminate waste from your body. Make no mistake, excess weight is waste.

▶ It's the by-product of all the artificial foods you eat that can't be built into healthy cells.

▶ It's the toxic debris from catabolism, the daily breaking down of cells that require energy to be eliminated.

▶ It's the waste stored in your colon, the fat stored in your tissues. You trim the fat from a steak before you grill it. You remove the fat from the chicken before you cook it. Because you see that fat as waste!

It is particularly relevant to call the excess fat on your body "waste" since it is in the fatty tissues that your body stores all the nonnutritious food additives, pharmaceuticals, contaminants, and pesticides you take in. Without energy, your body simply is unable to respond to your desire or efforts to eliminate that fat.

With adequate energy at its disposal, your body will automatically eliminate all excess waste, which means you will lose the weight you wish to lose. Your body has a built-in weight-loss mechanism, called the elimination system, which you can support or thwart. Learning how to support it as a lifestyle is like making sure you arrange for regular garbage collection from your home.

In the chapters that follow, you will learn tools for ongoing energy building and weight loss that you will be able to use for the rest of your life. Once you have these tools in mind, you'll know, without doubt, that your weight and health problems are finally in your control.

Inner cleanliness is so important to success in every area of your life. When you assist your elimination system to work for you, rather than thwart it, weight loss is easier. Productivity and creativity are enhanced. Relationships will improve. Spiritual growth is facilitated. How often have you heard it said, "Cleanliness is next to godliness"?

Inner Cleanliness:
The Secret to Natural Health

Let's take a moment to explore the idea of *inner* cleanliness, since it is not a commonly understood topic. Over the last hundred and fifty years in this country and around the world, great strides have been made in the area of sanitation. Many of the epidemics of infectious diseases that were killing us in that era, such as typhus, typhoid, cholera, smallpox, and consumption, were wiped out by improvements in sanitation. As we learned how to deal with sewage, as we began to understand the importance of ventilation, as we connected the filth and garbage around us to the diseases that were killing us, our health statistics began to improve. Then, as we discovered that spoiled food caused illness, we developed refrigeration, and our health statistics improved again.

Natural Health practitioners at the time were admonishing us to connect this idea of cleanliness to the inside of our bodies, but their voices were silenced before we were able to absorb the message. Instead we turned to admittedly toxic drugs, which *added* to our inner pollution rather than removed it.

When we failed to learn to apply sanitation to *inner* cleanliness, when we failed to realize that chemicals and contaminants in our air, water, and food—and the denaturing of our food supply—would only poison us, we found ourselves swapping the infectious diseases for newer maladies of our own making.

ONE OF THOSE MALADIES WAS EXCESS WEIGHT. By not properly caring for the inside of our bodies, we began to degenerate. And the weight tables began to climb to the record-breaking heights we see today.

In the name of cleanliness for the outside of our bodies, we bought Madison Avenue's claims for "better living through chemistry." We became fanatical about externals, spending billions of dollars every year on more-often-than-not *toxic* deodorants, mouthwashes, soaps, scrubs, salves, air fresheners, and cleaning agents. We failed to realize that much of the "unpleasantness" we were trying to mask was the result of a dirty inner body. A clean inner body is not saddled with excess weight. A clean inner body is not the breeding ground for disease. And a clean inner body is absolutely attainable. It is the result of a wholesome, nourishing, **clean** diet; regular exercise; and adequate rest. And . . . it is totally energy-dependent.

Meet Your Elimination System: Your Weight-Loss Buddy

Your natural cleaning system consists of your lungs, bladder, bowels, and skin, supported by your organs of filtration: the kidney, spleen, liver, and lymphatic system. In order for these organs to work for you as an ongoing cleansing and weight-loss mechanism, energy must be available in sufficient quantities, but, unfortunately, that is not usually the case.

Because of energy-robbing "foods" and energy-robbing stress, you are constantly undermining your elimination system. How does this work?

You see, this natural cleansing process of the body is the *one vital activity* from which energy can be *borrowed*. It's the *one vital activity* your body can *delay*. Your common sense will tell you that your body cannot take energy from the vital circulatory process. If your heart stops pumping, you're history. It can't delay respiration. You can survive only about six minutes without air. The same is true for digestion.

What do you think is the number-one drain on your personal energy supply? It's when food enters your stomach. Your body must deal with it. On the other hand, **elimination can and will be postponed if there is an energy deficit.** It's as if your body is saying, "Better dirty than dead."

You have seen this phenomenon at work in your life. If you are overworked, keeping late hours, or overeating, you will find that the likelihood of constipation is greater. When that happens, it's as if your body is speaking to you, saying, "Wait a minute, I'm so out of energy with all you're asking me to do, I don't have time to clean the house." Your body is cutting down on elimination because the energy supply simply isn't there for it. Waste is being retained rather than eliminated. And that's how you set the dreaded process in motion:

▶ Your jeans are too tight.

▶ You're loosening your belt.

▶ You're buying larger dresses.

A thwarted elimination system is the root cause of the unappealing situations that have you buying all those personal hygiene products. And it will go on and on, creating the distended abdomens so prevalent in our society, until the situation becomes life-threatening.

You may also notice that during times of stress—when you're not exercising, resting, or eating energy-building foods—your skin will break out. What you're seeing is toxic material coming out through the pores of the skin because it isn't being handled effectively by the colon and bladder. Your breath will be bad—it's coming out from the lungs.

Of course, you're continuously being deluged by snappy television commercials promising relief for these "commonly experienced" symptoms of waste retention by taking a dose of this or that drug. Many of these commercials even encourage you to eat what causes the problem or makes it worse, because a drug is available to mask the pain and other symptoms. To do so is to deny the Law of Cause and Effect. You cannot escape the repercussions of the harmful substances you put into your body. You cannot avoid a breakdown of the elimination system if you waste your energy in this fashion.

How Inner Cleanliness
Eludes Us

You clutter your body in two ways. The first is automatic. Remember your 50 trillion cells? That number is far, far greater than there are stars in our galaxy! You must remember that your cells are continuously being broken down, to the tune of billions every day. These worn-out cells are *toxic*. They must be eliminated. If you want to be in your best shape, you must *also* remember that it *takes* energy to eliminate dead cells. You have no control over this internal waste production, but you have every control over the energy to eliminate it. Waste production is involuntary, the nature of life on a microscopic scale, and it reflects the macrocosm of birth and death that takes place all around you.

In life, we make it a number-one priority to lovingly and carefully remove the dead from our physical presence. In our bodies, however, we unknowingly rob ourselves of the energy necessary to remove dead cells. Their remains float around in our bloodstreams as unspeakable toxicity.

Only you have control over the elimination of these dead, toxic cells. To keep dead cells from accumulating, you must embrace a lifestyle that provides your body with abundant energy. If you do, dead cells will be eliminated routinely, without a problem.

A second way waste is generated inside our bodies is by what we put into them. We burden ourselves with artificial sweeteners, fats, and "plastic" fat substitutes. We eat a steady diet of processed foods. We wolf down artificial ingredients as if our bodies are like the artificial "tin man." We take drugs at the drop of a hat. We're force-fed on pesticides, chemical additives, colorings and preservatives, food bacteria, and pollutants in water.

None of this stuff is the "food" Nature designed for our bodies. It is all purely and simply energy-draining. None of it can nourish, cleanse, or fuel. All of it must be eliminated. But since it is devitalized, unnatural, and poisonous to the body, it doesn't even generate the energy the body needs to eliminate it.

Here's How the Weight Piles On

It's a vicious cycle, a catch-22, and only you can change it. Until you do, your body has a defense mechanism that kicks in. It retains water (extra weight) to keep the toxic material in suspension and away from your vital organs. You get that puffy look. It stores toxins in your fat cells—your *toxic waste dumps*.

It loads up your fat cells and creates new ones to handle the onslaught of junk you're putting into your body. It also gives you alarm signals in the form of "general aches and pains." It keeps your defense, your immune system, in a constant state of mobilization. You think you're getting sick. You say you've caught something. Your doctor diagnoses that "something" and conveniently prescribes a toxic drug, while in reality all you're actually suffering from is "self-poisoning." The "quick fix" not only ignores the cause of your problem but may also add to it. And you're not getting any slimmer.

The choice of foods you make is the factor in cleanliness over which you have the *most* control, and the secret to being lean and clean is to know how to make food choices that build energy for elimination. What are these choices?

▶ Choose foods that are natural rather than processed. Foods such as fruits, vegetables, lean proteins, whole grains, and legumes that will give you energy rather than rob your energy.

▶ Choose water, herbal teas, and fresh vegetable or fruit juices as your beverages rather than sodas or caffeinated beverages. In addition to all the chemicals in sodas, they're carbonated with carbon dioxide, the poisonous gas our bodies continuously exhale.

If you lived in a house where you did not clean the floors, empty the garbage, and wash the linens, dishes, or windows, you could survive there, but what would it be like? Who in their right mind would ever want to live like that? Understand that you, like the majority of people, may be unknowingly allowing this neglect right inside your own body. How can you lose weight when you're so bogged down and clogged with toxicity? How can you ever feel really well?

Constipation:
The Root Cause of Our Ills

This is not a chic topic. Legions of authors aren't lining up to give you a heart-to-heart talk on this subject. Most likely this is not the part of the book you'll be discussing over lunch. However, if you want to be of normal weight, and truly and naturally healthy, you must face the fact that it will never happen if you're constipated.

Before we go any farther, allow us to clarify that we're not just talking about the standard definition of constipation, which has millions of Americans regularly taking harsh chemical laxatives or pounding down coffee first thing in the morning. We're talking about that and something much broader—and much more serious.

Natural Health pioneer Arnold Ehret taught us to picture the body as an intricate system of tubes, pipes, and filters, for that, in reality, is what it is. This tube/ pipe/filtration apparatus in-

"The percentage [of cardiovascular disease] is so high because virtually all American adults are at risk, unaware of silent heart blockages that may strike at any moment."
—Otis-Clapp Pharmaceuticals brochure, P.O. Box 9160, Canton, Mass. 02021

cludes your lymph system, arteries, veins, bronchial tubes, small intestine, and colon. The filters are your liver, lungs, and kidneys. If any of these are blocked, if they're not *squeaky clean*, then you're suffering from constipation.

Nearly all disease, including the undesired state of corpulence from which 60 million Americans are innocently suffering, is a form of either local or general constipation. This is a TRUTH that has been around for a century and is shared by practically every long-lived Natural Health pioneer and many doctors today. To quote Dr. Gabriel Cousens: "Many people think the phrase 'toxins in the body' is just some jargon of food faddists.

"Yet research over the last 100 years shows that these bowel toxins actually exist. Not only do they exist, but they have a tremendous negative impact on mental and physical well-being. Toxins usually come from a process called intestinal toxemia, an overgrowth of putrefactive intestinal bacteria in the small and large intestines. These toxins are then absorbed into the bloodstream and from there affect both our mental and physical functioning."[1]

In 1933, a twenty-five-year study of five thousand cases by Dr. Anthony Basler proved that intestinal toxemia is the most important factor in many diseases of the human body. At the time, Natural Health pioneers were telling us that the secret to health and a return to normal weight is to remove constipation. Arnold Ehret, author of *The Definite Cure of Chronic Constipation*, said that "chronic constipation is the worst and most common crime against life and humankind."

These are strong words, but we would have to agree with him. *It is a crime of the highest magnitude against your own well-being to allow your body to be internally blocked with waste.* Ehret spoke from his own personal experience with thousands of chronically diseased people. His conclusion echoes ours: The

---

[1]Gabriel Cousens. *Conscious Eating.* Santa Rosa, Calif.: Vision Books International, 1992, p. 101.

**The First Principle
of Natural Health and Weight Loss**

Keep the colon clean with fresh fruit, vegetables,
and high-fiber grains or legumes.

---

extent of your mental, spiritual, and physical capability is largely influenced by the condition of your digestive and eliminative organs.

▼
COLON HEALTH
Dr. Donald Schnell

Few of you will ever have the opportunity to perform an autopsy, but as a chiropractic student I had that opportunity, and it changed my life forever. Never in my wildest dreams could I have imagined what I saw in the twenty autopsies I was required to perform. The colon of every corpse I autopsied contained all manner of unwanted and toxic debris, from worms to petrified waste, encrusted on its walls. What a shock it was for me to see how *routinely* this eliminative organ had degenerated into a state of utter inefficiency. In my search for explanations for this sorry state of ill health, I consulted the work of Arnold Ehret. I found that he described the same situation.

In over two hundred and eighty-four autopsies Ehret performed, only twenty-eight colons were found to be free from hardened waste matter. I knew exactly what Ehret was referring to when he said, "As I stood looking at the colon . . . I expressed myself in wonder that anyone can live a week, much less for years, with such a cesspool of death and contagion always with him. The absorption of the deadly poison back into circulation cannot help but cause contagious diseases. . . . My experience during the past ten years has proven, by the rapid recovery of all diseases after the colon was cleansed, that in the colon itself lies the basic cause of almost all human ailments."[2]

---

[2]Arnold Ehret. *The Definite Cause of Chronic Constipation.* New York: American School of Naturopathy, 1922, p. 3.

From that point on, I never looked at the American potbelly in the same way again, and it *deeply* concerned me that no one was addressing this problem to the American people in candid enough terms to convince them to pay attention. I looked further for wisdom on how to bring the subject to light, to the works of Dr. N.W. Walker. In his book *Colon Health*, Dr. Walker includes graphic photos of the clogged colons typical of most people.

Instead of having a normal upside-down *U* shape, they are often in twisted positions, ballooned grotesquely with the burden of retained waste. Walker explains that any cooked or processed food can leave a coating on the inner walls of the colon that is much like plaster. The more processed it is, the more *unnatural*, the greater likelihood of residue being left behind. In the course of time, this coating may gradually increase in thickness until there's only a small opening through the center. In Dr. Walker's opinion, it is not unusual for people to be carrying around fifteen pounds of waste or more.[3]

▲

A Clean Machine Is a Lean Machine or If You Have a Potbelly, You've Gone to Waste

The heavier a person is, the greater the likelihood that stored waste will account for far more than fifteen pounds. The so-called potbelly, or beer belly, indicates an accumulation of waste matter blocking the intestines. We're not denying that many people also have an accumulation of fat in the abdominal area, but *trimming inches from the waste has a two-fold approach.* If that is your goal, cleansing the colon is a good place to start, especially if you're also interested in Natural Health and staying out of the hospital.

The late Carlson Wade, one of America's foremost medical and nutrition reporters, believed that auto-intoxication (which

---

[3]N.W. Walker. *Become Younger.* Prescott, Ariz.: Norwalk Press, 1978, p. 97.

is a clinical way of saying "your pipes, tubes, and filters are clogged") is responsible for causing the hospitalization of more people than any other group of disorders. Wade taught that inner cleansing can protect you from a broad spectrum of problems.[4] Our purpose in this book is to give you the easiest possible formula to ensure that this inner cleansing is efficient and ongoing, and weight loss is assured.

You run your brain, your nervous system, and every organ of your body on a continuous supply of nutrients within your bloodstream. Ideally, your bloodstream is pure and clean. But if your food is not digested properly, if you have acid indigestion, gas, flatulence, upset stomach, and other symptoms of impaired digestion, your bloodstream will not be clean. Discomfort after eating indicates that food is not breaking down efficiently. When this happens there is spoilage, fermentation of starches, and putrefaction of proteins.

You should know that this rotting mess must pass through your *entire* alimentary tract to be eliminated. (If you are unclear about exactly what your alimentary tract is, it extends from the point of entry of food at the mouth to the point of exit, at the other end.) Along the way, whatever nutrients have survived are absorbed into the bloodstream. Water is squeezed out and absorbed along with the poisonous toxic residue of spoiled food.

If every time you sat down to eat you were brought a plate half full of garbage and half full of food, all of which you were forced to eat, how long would you remain healthy? Theoretically, this is exactly what is going on whenever your digestion is impaired and food spoils in your body.

---

[4]Carlson Wade. *Inner Cleansing*. West Nyack, N.Y.: Parker Publishing Company, 1992, p. 226.

A New Concept:
The Many Forms of Constipation

Constipation of the colon itself is a disease, and a severe one, because of the insidious way it burdens your body with additional weight and pollutes your bloodstream. Common sense tells us it may be one of many conditions that leads to colon cancer, one of the major causes of suffering and death in this country.

▶ Constipation of the arteries leads to heart attacks and strokes, our number-one killer.

▶ Constipation of the lymph system sets up the conditions for several types of cancers, including breast cancer and lymphoma.

▶ Constipation of the lungs and bronchial area leads to lung cancer, pneumonia, asthma, allergies, and tuberculosis. If you smoke, take a clean glass and exhale a lungful of smoke into it. Notice the brown residue that coats the glass. Smoking and secondhand smoke constipate your lungs. As does air pollution.

Common sense will tell you:
Cleanliness and disease
do not go hand in hand.
When you rid the body of its "garbage,"
you're taking your first steps
toward weight loss and lasting health.

▶ Constipation of the liver and kidneys leads to nausea, kidney stones, gallstones, cirrhosis, hepatitis, and kidney failure. The liver is the most important organ for detoxification or cleansing. It is so vital to your health that you can live only a few hours without it. If it is clogged, the toxic poisons it would normally filter out back up into other parts of the body (in the same way that a clogged toilet will overflow). Excess weight and fat on the body insure a sluggish, fatty liver.

Fortunately, the liver is an organ that can be purified and regenerated, and one of the ways to start is with natural, healthful weight loss. Another piece of good news is that all of the above forms of constipation are lessened or eliminated when you embrace Natural Health.

It's Up to You:
Nobody Can Do It for You

You decide. Are you clean on the inside? Your body is always giving you clues. Here are the signs of inner pollution: excess weight, fatigue, gas, flatulence, belching, headaches, irritability, nervousness, nausea, depression, aches and pains, loss of memory and concentration, food cravings, insomnia, abdominal discomfort, menstrual problems, skin problems, poor appetite, coated tongue, bad breath, dark circles under the eyes, burning sensations in the stomach, and high blood pressure.

It is a tragic mistake to blame *any* of these common symptoms on causes outside your control. All can be remedied by a good inner housecleaning. And it is equally a mistake to assume that you are entirely to blame if you are experiencing any of these symptoms. You've probably never been told how to have an abundance of energy in your body and the inner cleanliness it will bring you. The secret lies in . . .

4

▼

Enzymes:
The Fountain of Youth

▼

*"In the 1900s, one hundred years after
the birth of modern scientific nutrition,
we find ourselves at an exciting juncture.
A missing link in our understanding
of the life-giving properties of food
is being illuminated by the increasing acceptance
of the critical role of food-based enzymes
for health and longevity."*

—VICTOR P. KULVINSKAS,
SURVIVAL INTO THE 21ST CENTURY

Enzymes are the life action in every living thing. They are the substances that carry life force. Just as the photon is the measure of *light*, the enzyme is the measure of *life*. Life is activity, and enzymes are responsible for all the activity that takes place in your body and in every other living thing.

The word *enzyme* comes from the Greek word *enzymas*, which means "to ferment" or "to cause a change." Enzymes are the substances that cause an apple or a peach to ripen and eventually rot. If you place a green banana on your windowsill for a few days, you can watch it turn yellow, develop brown speckles, and then finally turn black. That is enzyme activity. A piece of raw chicken left on the same windowsill will begin to have an unpalatable odor. Enzymes are breaking down the flesh. It is decomposing. Inside your body, the enzymes in the fruit *predigest* it before the enzymes in your body finish off the task.

Natural Health pioneer Dr. Edward Howell, who began his research in the 1930s, taught us that the only workers in the body are enzymes. From Howell we learn that vitamins, minerals, fats, carbohydrates, and proteins cannot work. Only enzymes are designed to work. Although there is a natural symbiotic relationship between enzymes, proteins, and minerals in particular, without enzymes none of these can do anything. Only enzymes *do*.

Nature's Labor Force

Enzymes are needed for every chemical and biological reaction that occurs in your body. You can't run, walk, breathe, or blink without enzymes. You can't see or hear, think, move a muscle, or have sex without them. You can't digest your food, repair your cells, or cleanse your body without enzyme activity. The building of your blood, bone, and skin requires them. You can't keep your bloodstream clean without them. Your defense system depends on enzymes—and NOTHING ELSE—to attack invaders, mop up chemical poisons and contaminants, and scavenge up the cellular debris produced every day by the process of metabolism.

Remember the millions of cells that break down routinely every day in your body. As we said in the preceding chapter, those cells are *toxic*. They must be eliminated by enzymes as quickly as they are generated if you are to stand a chance of being of normal weight and health. So what do you think happens when you are low in enzymes? Right. Your body stores waste and weight. You get sick. Do you ever have an achy day or feel as if your mind is in a fog? Or maybe you just feel "slowed down"? That is a low-enzyme day.

Energy is the currency in your body, and it is the ultimate commodity for Natural Health and weight loss. Every day your body must manufacture a quantity of energy in your cells equal to your body weight. In every aspect of that process, enzymes *must* be present.

--- ᚷᚫᚹ ---

Enzymes are Nature's workers.
They are your body's labor force.

--- ᚷᚫᚹ ---

Three thousand enzymes have been discovered in the human body; in the arteries alone there are ninety-eight enzymes carrying out specific tasks. It has been estimated that each cell in the liver contains at least *fifty different enzymes* that perform their work a million times a second. In a single minute, one enzyme can be involved in *thirty-six million* biochemical reactions. Every cell in your body produces enzymes, but . . . you must know that **the supply of enzymes in your body is *not* unlimited.**

Your Personal Enzyme Story

Where do the enzymes in your body come from? You inherit a certain ability to manufacture enzymes at birth. This is called your Enzyme Capacity, and it is unique for each individual. Your Enzyme Capacity is a finite quantity of energy factors that must last a lifetime.

As you get older, your body's ability to produce enzymes dwindles. It's as if you inherited a certain amount of money at birth. If you were constantly squandering it throughout your early years, you would be short-changed when you needed it most in midlife and your senior years. Conservation of enzymes is one of the keys to Natural Health and weight loss. Respecting your enzymes will go a long way toward ensuring fitness and a longer, healthier life. So look at your Enzyme Capacity as an *enzyme savings account.* The less you withdraw, the more you have.

All foods as Nature produces them, either in the field or orchard, and even in the barnyard or ocean, in their *living* state, contain enzymes. In other words, food, in its natural, raw state, carries with it the enzymes you need to predigest it.

"So, if you're telling me I need to eat more raw food, does that include a tuna fish sandwich?" someone always asks. "I don't have to cook that."

No, it doesn't. You don't have to cook it, but others do before it gets to you.

All fresh fruits and vegetables are particularly rich in enzymes. When you eat them in their natural state, you take a tremendous burden off your own enzyme supply. The more raw foods you eat, the fewer withdrawals you take from your enzyme savings accounts. *Why is this important? Because . . . the digestion of food requires more enzymes than any other single process of your body.*

The Asians learned this secret thousands of years ago, when they began to use enzymes to predigest soybeans, so that important protein source would be more easily digestible. Soy milk, tofu, tempeh, and miso are soy products that are far easier to digest than the original soybean from which they are produced. As protein sources, they tax your body's enzyme supply far less than animal proteins because they are predigested.

You're Killing Your Enzymes

Unfortunately, all food enzymes, LIKE ALL OTHER LIVING THINGS, begin to die at temperatures between 118 and 160 degrees. Therefore, when you continually eat cooked food, you are making withdrawals from your body's personal enzyme savings account. Enzymes are destroyed by all cooking or processing of food. In other words, whether you bake, boil, steam, broil, microwave, stew, or grill, you will destroy the enzymes in your food. If your foods are pasteurized, frozen, canned, or sterilized, the enzymes will have been destroyed.

Enzymes and Weight Loss

Dr. Edward Howell was one of the first scientists to understand the link between the enzymes in food and our health. A medical doctor, Howell had no interest in surgery or drugs but was convinced that the field of Natural Health had answers that were being overlooked by conventional medicine. He aligned himself with the famous naturopathic physician Dr. Henry Lindlahr and worked at the Lindlahr Sanitarium for over six years. It was at the sanitarium where he witnessed Lindlahr's enormous success in restoring countless patients to glowing health and *normal weight.*

What was Lindlahr's secret? Dr. Howell felt it was *some ingredient* in the raw food regimen Lindlahr administered to his patients. When Howell went into his own private practice for the treatment of obesity and chronic ailments by nutritional means, he was determined to isolate the magic ingredient in the uncooked natural foods Lindlahr was using. He discovered it was *enzymes.* Howell determined that the only nutritional factor always present in uncooked foods and never present in cooked foods was enzymes. He realized that these "units of life energy," the *labor force,* that was bringing about so much improvement in his patients' health, was destroyed in temperatures over 118 degrees. He understood that this made enzymes *much more sensitive* to heat than vitamins and minerals.

Before we proceed, we want you to understand clearly that we don't expect you to be living on a raw food diet. But if you want to lose excess weight and increase your energy, we *do* encourage you to eat far more live food than you may be eating

▼

Mineral Supplements

In the 1930s, the U.S. government released studies proving the depletion of minerals in our topsoil. Today, the situation is far worse. Our nonorganic produce is stimulated to grow with fertilizers that do not replace minerals in the soil. According to government statistics, a tomato today has 50 percent fewer minerals than fifty years ago.

Soils provide the minerals necessary for plant development. Plants serve as food for the animals that assimilate them. Then, we eat the meat. The minerals then act as co-vitamins and co-enzymes in our metabolism. Without the proper minerals, our bodies cannot fully absorb nutrients and eliminate waste.

Therefore, in the pursuit of Natural Health, we now *must* supplement the minerals in our diets. But what kind are most helpful? Most mineral supplements—for example, calcium supplements from ground oyster shells—can be only minimally assimilated by your body (as little as 5 percent). A relatively recent breakthrough technology provides plant minerals in colloidal form that can be assimilated up to 100 percent.

We call such colloidal minerals "tonics," and we, and thousands like us, drink them every day to ensure the highest quality of health. They are available at your natural food store.

A paper in the April 12, 1995, issue of the *Journal of the American Medical Association* detailed the results of a moderately large, very long-term epidemiological study of dietary habits and stroke. Using eight hundred males participating in the Framington Study, doctors at Harvard Medical School assessed dietary intake of fruits and vegetables over a twenty-year period.

The results are no surprise: The (age adjusted) risk of stroke decreased with increasing consumption of fruits and vegetables.

▲

now. Fifty percent of Americans don't eat even one piece of fruit a day.[1] Of course, you are aware that nearly everyone in our country is subsisting on a predominantly cooked food diet, which is a diet totally lacking in enzymes.

---

[1]*Muscular Development*, December 1995, p. 34.

Of all the species on earth, we are the *only* one to cook our food. And we're enzyme deficient because of it. And we're the only species, with the exception of animals kept as pets, to suffer from obesity and the degenerative diseases.

Enzymes and Your Health

The significance of enzymes in the diet was first discovered in a ten-year study by Dr. Francis Pottenger in the 1920s. Over the ten-year period, Pottenger fed nine hundred cats an enzyme-rich diet of fresh raw meat and raw milk and found these cats maintained their health and vitality throughout several generations. A second group of cats was fed a diet of cooked meat and pasteurized milk.

In *Food Enzymes: The Missing Link to Radiant Health*, Dr. Humbart Santillo reports: "Those on cooked food developed our modern ailments: heart, kidney, and thyroid disease; pneumonia; paralysis; loss of teeth; difficulty in labor; diminished or perverted sexual interest; diarrhea; and irritability. Liver impairment on cooked protein was progressive, the bile in the stool becoming so toxic that even weeds refused to grow in soil fertilized by the cat's excrement. The first generation of kittens were sick and abnormal; the second generation were often born dead or diseased; by the third generation, the mother was sterile."[2] Pottenger's study supports the idea that enzymes are the vital factor to health and longevity in raw food that cannot be found in cooked food.

Enzymes for Prevention

How serious is this drain on our enzyme capacity caused by diets of mostly cooked foods? We believe it is one of the para-

---

[2]Humbart Santillo. *Food Enzymes: The Missing Link to Radiant Health.* Prescott, Ariz.: Hohm Press, 1991, p. 35.

mount causes of overweight, premature aging, and early death. We also believe that it is the underlying cause of almost all degenerative diseases.

Many scientists agree. Dr. Howell certainly did. And according to Drs. D. A. Lopez, R.M. Williams, and M. Miehlke, authors of *Enzymes: The Fountain of Life*: "Some scientists feel this shortfall in metabolic enzymes contributes to some of our modern society diseases, such as degenerative disorders (osteoarthritis, emphysema, osteoporosis, gastrointestinal disorders, Alzheimer's, etc.) and to some autoaggressive diseases (collagen vascular diseases such as rheumatoid arthritis, lupus, scleroderma, etc.) and to cancer."[3]

▼

The word *Eskimo*, derived from a Native American Indian language, means "he who eats food raw." Eskimos predigest their fish by burying it live in ice, and not eating it until it ages. The enzymes in the live tissues of the fish begin to break it down. When the Eskimos eat the fish in this state, it is called "high fish," because it gives them more strength and endurance than fish that is caught and eaten immediately.[4]

Eskimos who consume ten pounds of raw meat and blubber daily have practically no signs of clogged arteries. That's because the enzyme lipase in the live food they are eating breaks down the fat and aids in the prevention of circulatory diseases.

In 1926, Dr. William A. Thomas of the MacMillan Arctic Expedition wrote: "Eskimos live on an exclusively meat and fish diet, all usually and preferably eaten in the raw. There was no unusual prevalence of renal (kidney) and vascular (circulatory) disease. However, the Eskimos that began living mostly on cooked foods [had a change in health] . . . Cancer and heart disease appeared and their longevity was reduced 50 percent."[5]

▲

---

[3]D. A. Lopez, R. M. Williams, and M. Miehlke. *Enzymes: The Fountain of Life.* Charleston, S.C.: Neville Press, 1994.

[4]Santillo. *Food Enzymes*, p. 29.

[5]Victor P. Kulvinskas. *Don't Dine Without Enzymes.* Hot Springs, Ark.: L.O.V.E. Foods, Inc., 1994, pp. 20–21.

In other words, the metabolic inefficiency that results from eating enzyme-deficient meals may be laying the groundwork for cancer, coronary heart disease, diabetes, and many other chronic diseases. Tragically, this state of enzyme deficiency exists in the majority of persons on the Standard American Diet (S.A.D.).

How Much Do You Expect from Your Body?

It makes such common sense. If your body is overburdened by a cooked and processed food diet, struggling to supply the many enzymes needed for digestion, it must curtail the production of enzymes for other purposes. What do you think happens to you if your enzymes are forced to leave their highly specialized work sites to answer the body's call for digestive enzymes? If they are taken from your immune system, it is similar to taking nuclear physicists from their laboratories and asking them to sweep the streets!

When enzymes are being allocated constantly for digestion, how can the body also keep producing an adequate supply to run your brain, heart, kidneys, lungs, muscles, defense or immune system, and all the other organs and tissues? This "borrowing" of enzymes from other vital body systems to service the digestive tract sets up a competition for enzymes among the various organs and tissues. This weakens the functioning of these vital systems and keeps you from feeling at your highest level of health.

Cooked Food Is a Costly Choice

As far back as the 1930s, Dr. Paul Kouchakoff demonstrated that there is an increase in white blood cells after eating cooked food. These blood cells, called leucocytes, are needed to transport enzymes to the digestive tract. Kouchakoff also showed that after a live food meal, there is no noticeable increase in white blood cells.[6]

The increase in leucocytes can be easily explained. They contain enzymes that are used by your body to scavenge foreign proteins and other invaders in the blood. These important workers are being transported to aid in digestion as if the cooked food were poison, leaving you undefended from infection and disease and simultaneously depleting your enzyme capacity.

If you look up *leucocytosis*, which is what this process is called, in Dorland's Medical Dictionary, you will find that, in a nutshell, it means your white blood cell count is up, and something is wrong. And all you've done is eaten a cooked meal. Typically, white blood cell counts are high during infections or some form of medical pathology. When you are acutely ill, and your body is marshaling its enzymes to fight off the problem, your enzyme count will be high. On the other hand, if the disease lingers and becomes chronic, the enzyme levels in your blood will be lower and lower as you deplete your supply, fighting the illness. It's just like what happens when you become chronically ill. When you're hospitalized, your life savings are gobbled up little by little, by modern medical technology and the exorbitant fees it requires.

We're Skimping on Life

There is overwhelming evidence, literally thousands of scientific documents, indicating that humans are suffering from food enzyme deficiency—which means we're skimping on the food that gives us life! Human beings have the lowest levels of starch-

---

[6]Paul Kouchakoff. "The Influence of Food Cooking on the Blood Formula of Man." Lausanne, Switzerland: Institute of Clinical Chemistry, 1930.

digesting enzymes in their blood than any other creature. We also have the highest levels of these enzymes in our urine. What this indicates is that our starch-digesting enzymes are being used up! These low enzyme levels are not due to a peculiarity of our species. Instead, they are the direct result of our excessive consumption of starch.[7]

There's no way we can argue that! We routinely reach for bread, pasta, chips, cookies, french fries, cake, pie, and starchy snacks of all kinds. These starchy foods are relatively new to our species. We've been accustomed to eating meat, raw fruits, and vegetables from the moment we learned to walk upright and swing a club, but the quantity and variety of starches that are now the focus of our diet have only been available for less than two hundred years. Primitive men and women did not even have wheat, let alone donuts!

The massive intake of refined carbohydrates, such as white sugar and white flour products, has been going on for less than a century. Our bodies can't handle it; it's not recognized as *food*. Therefore, our starch-digesting enzymes are depleting rapidly and are thus showing up in our urine.

Look at what's happened to us since we've stopped eating "an apple a day"! Medical doctors are noting that in a number of chronic ailments, such as allergies, skin disease, diabetes, and even cancer, there are decreased enzyme levels. And since we've already pointed out that it takes enzymes to build energy, how are you going to feel any pep if you're enzyme deficient? Since weight loss requires energy as well, how are you going to lose those extra pounds?

Just as there are acceptable levels of white blood cells, there are acceptable levels of enzymes. With obesity, Dr. Howell observed that food enzyme deficiency was an important cause in adults and children. In his widely read book, *Enzyme Nutrition*, he cites evidence indicating that cooked, enzyme-deficient diets contribute to a pathological deviation of size in the pituitary

---

[7]Ibid., *Healthview Newsletter*.

gland and to changes in its appearance.[8] This is significant if you are trying to lose weight. Whether you are burning fat or storing it depends on the condition of your pituitary gland.

A cooked food diet will also ensure an enlarged pancreas. Since there are no food enzymes in all the cooked food you are eating to carry out the job of predigestion, the pancreas must increase in size to provide more internal enzymes to get the job done. It's a classic case of *enzyme undernutrition*. While the call for enzymes to digest your cooked food meals is unrelenting, the rest of your body's systems, robbed of their metabolic enzymes, are simply wearing out.

Enlarged glands and organs are not to be ignored. We take the condition lightly because they are under our skin and cannot, for the most part, be seen. But consider the enlarged thyroid gland, which is called a goiter. In addition to being debilitating, it is ugly—something most of us would wish to avoid at all costs. Enlarged kidneys, livers, or spleens are equally serious. Please don't make the mistake of taking an enlarged pancreas lightly. In autopsies of cancer victims, such a condition is routinely discovered. An oversized organ is overworked.

It would probably not surprise you to hear that the enlarged pancreas is practically a universal finding today in human beings—because . . . we're not eating enough raw food! Are you anxious at this point to have your enzymes used up faster? We hope, by now, your answer is a resounding "NO!"

Remember the Good Old Days?

Remember how you used to eat in your teens? A few hours after a breakfast of bacon and eggs, cereal and toast, and a glass of milk, you would stop in at the local drive-in for a double cheeseburger, fries, and a milk shake. Then you went to the

---

[8]Edward Howell. *Enzyme Nutrition.* Wayne, N.J.: Avery Publishing Group, 1985, p. 106.

movies or the amusement park and ate popcorn, cotton candy, ice cream, a chocolate bar, and a Coke; and you arrived home just in time to enjoy two helpings of fried chicken, mashed potatoes and gravy, some canned corn, several glasses of milk, and two slices of chocolate cake or apple pie for dinner.

That's how most young people are able to eat—without putting on an inch or gaining a pound—because during the teenage years most enzyme accounts are full. Full accounts can handle teenage eating.

Research has proved that you have far greater quantities of enzymes in your body in your youth than when you are older. You have experienced the truth of this in your own life, and you have seen it at work, over and over, in the lives of those around you.

When did you first begin to notice you couldn't eat like that anymore, at least not without experiencing some distress or weight gain? In *The Secret of Life—Enzymes*, Dr. James B. Sumner, Nobel laureate and professor of biochemistry at Cornell University, wrote that the "getting old" feeling after forty— what we call the middle-age "blahs," those years of weight gain—are due to reduced enzyme levels in the body, the onset of enzyme depletion, and the dwindling of your Enzyme Capacity.

By the time you enter your senior years, you fully accept that you "can't eat what you used to" and you make a lifestyle of "watching your diet" and taking drugs for stomach pain and other symptoms of poor digestion. You are running out of enzymes, directly experiencing the truth of your dwindling ability to produce enzymes. The life enzymes carry is abundant in youth. When the bloodstreams of newborns are analyzed and compared to those of the elderly, there is little difference in the relative amounts of vitamins and minerals. The enzyme levels are an entirely different story: There are over one hundred times more enzymes in newborns than in the elderly.[9]

---

[9]Kulvinskas. *Don't Dine Without Enzymes*, p. 14.

---

*You are not just what you eat;
you are what you digest and assimilate!*

A Live Meal a Day
Keeps Those Extra Pounds Away

If you are trying to lose weight, it is important to know that, when animals in laboratory studies are placed on cooked diets they are always heavier than animals on raw food diets, even though the caloric levels of the food are equal. Raw foods help to normalize body weight because of their high enzyme content. Farmers have proved this by feeding cooked potatoes to hogs to produce rapid weight gain and therefore ensure a higher market price.[10]

When enzymes and energy are conserved, your body can put that extra vitality toward a major priority: the lightening of the burden on your heart. Your heart is designed to handle your normal body weight. Excess weight causes it to strain, as it is forced to pump blood into excess pounds of flesh it is not intended to handle. In fact, for every ten pounds of excess weight, your heart is forced to pump blood through an additional seven hundred miles of capillaries.

Dr. Howell noticed in his work at the Lindlahr Sanitarium that it was impossible for people to gain weight on enzyme-rich live foods, regardless of the caloric content of the foods. In our work in the Natural Health field over the past decades, we have always been trimmer and more energetic whenever we have

---

[10]Santillo. *Food Enzymes*, p. 26.

lived uniquely on live food, and we also have proven to our-selves repeatedly that it is the amount of live food we eat in proportion to the cooked food we eat that determines our level of health. Those who have been most motivated using FITON-ICS—and have focused more heavily on fresh fruits, vegetables, and their juices—have lost the most weight.

▼

Lipase: A Key Enzyme for Weight Loss

Dr. Gabriel Cousens reports on research done at Tufts Medical School: "In 100 percent of the cases of obesity studied, all of the people had lipase deficiencies. The implication was that they had a decreased ability to assimilate fat properly. The fat ended up being stored as fatty tissue, rather than being broken down."[11] Lipase is the enzyme that breaks down fats; it is found naturally in all high-fat *live* foods. Lipase prevents the fat we consume from being stored as fatty tissue.

Dr. Humbart Santillo writes: "At Stanford University, investiga-tions showed that lipase was deficient in patients who had hardening of the arteries. The more advanced the case, the more a deficiency in enzymes was found. When lipase was given to patients with slow fat metabolism and blood fat problems, there was an immediate improve-ment in fat metabolism."[12]

It was frequently asked why avocados were recommended in FIT FOR LIFE when they're so high in fat. The reason they became practi-cally a staple for millions of readers is due to the lipase they contain. In moderation, the fat in an avocado is one of the *best* fats you can eat because it carries with it its own digestive "team" of lipase enzymes! It can be so efficiently digested, your body can use it rather than store it.

▲

The success of FIT FOR LIFE can be largely traced to the fact that readers were encouraged to include fruits and vegetables

[11]Gabriel Cousens. *Conscious Eating.* Santa Rosa, Calif.: Vision Books Interna-tional, 1992, p. 341.
[12]Santillo. *Food Enzymes,* p. 28.

in their diets in a 70 percent ratio to the other foods they were eating. Once again, to be absolutely clear, we are not advocating that you eat more live food than you are comfortable eating. And we would never ask you, nor would we suggest, that you begin to forgo all the wonderful cooked food meals you enjoy. The strategy we will give you to "have your cake and eat it too" is to simply add more live food to your daily meal planning. This is an integral part of FITONICS, and it won't be difficult to embrace.

The Second Principle
of Natural Health and Weight Loss

To keep enzyme supplies high and energy abundant, and to support weight loss, eat one live food meal every day, consisting solely of fresh fruits or vegetables.

The success of FIT FOR LIFE proved to us that the most effective way to shed excess weight is to focus on fruit rather than on any other food in the morning. We do this religiously. Have a fruit breakfast in the form of juice, a "tonic," or a fruit plate or salad. Our favorite breakfast, the FIT-TONIC, is a synergistic blend of fruit juice and fruit with highly nutritious and energizing ingredients. It's our secret antiaging and energy formula, full of so many enzymes and nutrients that it curbs an appetite for hours. We find our FIT-TONIC to be the perfect answer for those who want the most from the foods they eat with the least amount of time and energy expended.

If you have difficulty tolerating large quantities of fruit, be sure you have at least a banana. Make sure your live meal is a large vegetable salad at lunch or dinner.

Many experts argue that a good, solid breakfast is the key meal of the day. Judith Wurtman, Ph.D., a research scientist at MIT, says, "If the kitchen isn't on your morning map, take heart; eating within three hours of waking up will deliver the breakfast boost. Having fresh fruit in some form keeps your blood sugar levels even until you have time to eat more heavily."[13]

If you live in a cold climate and feel the need for warm food, or if you are one of those people who simple *must* eat a substantial meal in the morning, have your fruit meal at lunch or dinner. If you choose to have a cooked meal at breakfast and at supper, eat only live food, fruit, and/or a salad at lunch.

Our years of experience have proved to us that, if weight loss and energy are your goals, the fruit-in-the-morning choice will give you the best results most of the time. Here's why:

When you go to sleep at night, your body is still converting what you have eaten in the evening to usable energy. You awaken in the morning with that energy in reserve and at your disposal. If you eat a heavy meal, most of your energy will go to digesting that meal. As a result, you will feel your energy drop and will need the habitual coffee break. Having fruit as your first meal of the day gives you a chance to burn the stored energy from your evening meal, it adds quick energy to your bloodstream, and it affords a substantial saving of enzymes. As you begin to form this habit, be sure you eat plenty of fruit. Have a large tonic or fruit salad and take as many morning fruit "breaks" as you need to feel satisfied.

---

[13]Judith Wurtman. *Managing Your Mind and Mood Through Food*. New York: HarperCollins, 1987.

A Tool, Not a Rule

It is important for you to understand one key to your live meal guideline in the morning: Have it whenever you can, but if you need a heavier breakfast, have your tonic or fruit first before the other foods you may want. In cold weather, you may crave a bowl of hot oatmeal, or a bowl of high-fiber cereal. If you are going on a long hike or if your evening meal the night before was unusually light, you may want a heartier breakfast. Once in a while, you may take a morning "break" and have a full brunch. You see, this is not a *law* we are laying down for you, but rather a guiding principle you can use as much or as little as you wish, depending on your goals.

Since enzyme-rich live meals add **LIFE** to your body, you'll soon find out how much fun they add to your life. As you eat more live food, delicious "tonics," or meals of fresh fruits and vegetables, you'll feel lighter, more energetic, and you'll begin to notice that you look better. Your weight will start to drop and your digestion will improve. You may notice that you are free of some of the aches and pains you were beginning to accept as just being "part of life." You'll begin to "crave" exercise, as the added life force courses through your veins.

And, as an added bonus to all the good you will be doing for yourself, you will be able to take advantage of miraculous breakthroughs in enzyme technology through . . .

5

▼

Enzyme Supplementation

▼

New Technology Jeopardizes the American Diet

Dr. Howell and other Natural Health pioneers were lone voices in a wilderness of enzyme ignorance. Like his colleagues, Howell agonized over a solution to the cooked food diet of the 1930s which was causing such a breakdown in health. He knew that foods had to be cooked to be canned and realized that when canned food became the hot new convenience item on the grocer's shelves, American enzyme intake would suffer a serious blow. Suddenly, Dr. Howell was witnessing a dramatic drop in the health of our population.

But Dr. Howell knew his patients wouldn't rush to give up cooked food or the new canned foods. Imagine how *convenient* these foods appeared to the American consumer. For the first time ever, Americans could eat corn or peas out of season. The American housewife no longer had to lug home a bag of apples if she wanted to make applesauce. The runaway withdrawals from our enzyme savings accounts were about to begin. As canned foods became more and more popular, signs of enzyme deficiencies and degeneration began to climb, and the American family began to suffer.

Out of the Frying Pan, into the Fire

As consumers enthusiastically embraced canned food as superior to fresh food, they were never told it was *deficient*, only that it was more *convenient*. We live out this same scenario today—in fact, a worse scenario. Today, we have not only canned foods but also a myriad of other processed foods that, albeit convenient, steal the enzymes from our food and rob the health from our lives.

Enzymes are responsible for ripening your food so you will eat it when it is ready for eating, the way Mother Nature intended.

For this reason, enzymes and the Life Force they carry are obviously the enemies of the food industry, which understandably aims for the longest possible shelf life to increase profits. Through lengthy storage and shipping practices, intensive use of chemical fertilizers and pesticides, premature harvesting, refining, pasteurization, biogenetic engineering, sterilization, and food irradiation, the enzymes in food are destroyed. The life in the food is removed so it can sit on the shelf, tasteless but looking pretty, long after it should have been thrown away.

The Breakthrough

Can you imagine how the health picture in this country, how your health and that of your loved ones, could improve if you could just add back the enzymes the processors have removed; in other words, add a good deal of supplemental enzymes to every cooked meal.

And you can! Food enzymes are now available in capsule form. These supplemental enzymes have the same effect in your body as the enzymes in live foods. You can now stop the drain on your body's enzyme capacity. You can make deposits to your enzyme savings account by taking enzyme supplements with every cooked meal.

We take them at every meal. And hundreds of thousands of people on the road to Natural Health do the same. Let's be clear about the benefits. The enzyme supplements you take will do much of the work of predigesting the enzyme-deficient cooked food you are eating. This single act, coupled with the live food meals you eat every day, and the occasional Funday you give yourself, will increase your enzyme "net worth" over time, allowing for an adequate enzyme labor force to be available for all the life-sustaining processes in your body.

Enzymes in Supplement Form

With special technology, enzymes are cultured from various forms of live food sources and are then low-temperature dried. The most widely available are papain and bromelaine (from papaya and pineapple), which specifically help predigest proteins. These are chewable tablets that are taken directly after a meal. A second type of plant enzyme is grown on aspergillus, a cultivation medium that has a many-thousand-year history in Asia in the production of tofu, miso, and other soy products. This type is helpful in the digestion of *any* cooked food you eat.

How Enzyme Supplements Work

When you begin to chew your food, digestion begins in your mouth where ptyalin, a salivary digestive juice, begins the breakdown of carbohydrates. Your food then passes into the upper or cardiac portion of your stomach,[1] where there is low acid secretion and a very limited amount of churning action.

In his *Theory of Enzyme Potential,* Dr. Howell called this cardiac part of your stomach the "Food Enzyme" stomach, because this is where the enzymes in live food and the plant enzyme supplements you take *with* cooked food work to predigest the food you have eaten.

This predigestion opportunity lessens the burden normally placed on the pancreas, as it is routinely required to convert enzymes from all the "work sites" in the rest of your body (the metabolic enzymes) for digestion. (If you have not taken any food enzyme supplements with your meal, and if your food is entirely cooked and therefore enzyme deficient, there will be far less predigestive activity since only the ptyalin from your saliva will be at work on the initial breakdown of carbohydrates.) Meanwhile, what about predigestion of the proteins and fats?

Dr. Howell found that while food enzymes and ptyalin work on the predigestion of your food in the "Food Enzyme" stomach, the lower portion of your stomach, the pyloric stomach, remains relatively inactive when you first eat, and even acid secretion there is minimal for at least thirty to sixty minutes.

Medical Texts Support the Theory

Medical students learn about the distinct activity in the two parts of the stomach in a standard medical textbook called

---

[1]Called "cardiac" because it is the portion of the stomach closest to the heart.

Gray's Anatomy, but we believe this important aspect of human digestion is seriously overlooked in the traditional medical understanding, which views the stomach as one container, as if it were a sack. What we are describing is, in fact, a perfectly logical aspect of Nature's design, which allows for the enzymes in the food you eat (or the supplements you take) to do their work before the stomach is required to secrete digestive acids and additional enzymes to finish the job.

Common sense tells you: *The more predigestion that occurs, the less work your pancreas will have to do later.* Thus, the burden on your pancreas is lightened and the drain from your enzyme savings account is lessened.

When this thirty-to-sixty-minute predigestion phase has elapsed, the food enters the lower portion of your stomach, where the necessary acid and enzymes are being secreted to further the digestive breakdown of your meal. Here, your stomach works hard to digest the proteins you have eaten, particularly if they are animal proteins. At this point, as acidity levels rise, the plant-based food enzymes are inactivated. They will be reactivated in your small intestine, where they can continue to aid your body's own pancreatic enzymes in the digestive process.

Many nutritionists and medical doctors who have not adequately studied enzymes for nutrition believe that plant enzymes are destroyed by stomach acid and are therefore of little or no value. This is the old party line in medicine, which is giving way to an entirely new understanding based on research both abroad and in our country. New research, specifically in Europe and Japan, is fostering a new model that enzymes are inactivated (not destroyed) in the stomach and are reactivated in the small intestine.[2] Let us remind you, the Japanese and most European countries have now bypassed the United States in longevity.

---

[2]Humbart Santillo. *Food Enzymes: The Missing Link to Radiant Health.* Prescott, Ariz.: Hohm Press, 1987, p. 12.

The "Pac-Man" Effect

There is evidence that enzyme supplements may be of benefit even when taken *between* meals. Without food to predigest, they can then be added to your enzyme account as "volunteer workers," tiny scavenging "Pac-men," in your bloodstream. Here again, the current **American** scientific theory is that no enzyme, including a supplement, survives stomach acid (since enzymes are encased in a protein coat and stomach acid digests proteins). Keep in mind, however, that in the United States, we lag far behind Germany and other European countries, as well as Japan, in our enzyme research and application for therapy. Are American scientists forgetting that when babies are born, they depend on mother's milk to provide them with the **enzymes** necessary for their immune systems? There is no scientific dispute whatsoever that these enzymes survive the acid in the baby's stomach and are absorbed through the small intestine into the bloodstream.

In *Enzyme Therapy*, two leading enzyme researchers in Germany, Dr. Max Wolf and Dr. Karl Ransberger, reported tagging certain enzymes with radioactive dye to see if these enzymes could be traced in the bloodstream. The tagged enzymes were found in the liver, spleen, kidneys, heart, lungs, duodenum, and urine.[3]

The significance of the discovery that we can *add* to our own enzyme bank cannot be overemphasized. This is a tremendous breakthrough. Think for a moment of the benefit to your health and longevity when enzymes, not used up in digestion, end up as workers in your bloodstream!

Enzyme products are not a new idea with food manufacturers. The popular enzyme supplement Beano, with sales in the billions of dollars, works on breaking down certain gas-forming

[3]Ibid., p. 9.

sugars in beans. But beans are so much more than just the sugars. Beano lacks enzyme activity to break down the concentrated proteins that beans contain.

An enzyme-supplemented dairy product, Lactaid, helps people who are unable to digest the milk sugar in dairy products. Raw milk is full of enzymes that enable the human body to digest it, but the pasteurization process removes them. Lactaid, ironically, is the dairy industry's attempt to replace crucial nutrients that *they themselves removed.*

Full-Spectrum Enzymes

As a result of a growing awareness and concern regarding the missing enzymes in our diets, new breakthroughs in enzyme supplementation allow us to use enzymes that aid digestion of not only sugars, but proteins, fats, and carbohydrates as well. In other words, they contain protease (for proteins), lipase (for fats), and amylase (for carbohydrates). This represents a crucial development essential to the FITONICS lifestyle. Enzyme supplements promote good digestion, good health, and thus, ultimately, facilitate weight loss. Again, it's common sense. As these enzymes expedite digestion, absorption, and assimilation, you're getting "more bang for your buck" when you eat. The hypothalamus, which tells you if you're hungry or full, registers nourishment rather than "more nutrients, please," and you tend to eat less. The feeling that you need to eat all the time comes to a halt.

According to John Naisbitt, author of *Megatrends,* "Biology will be to the 21st Century what physics and chemistry were to this century. . . . The main area of interest will be the production of enzymes. . . ."

Enzymes Cross the Atlantic

In 1962, the American Medical Association predicted that in the future, *enzymes* would be the most promising word in research. That future is NOW! Enzymes in supplement form are presently available for a wide variety of applications. The most important for the purposes of this book is their use for *effective digestion* and *maximum nutrient absorption* which result in good health.

Success with Enzymes in Europe

Research that has been done in Europe is frequently not translated into English and is therefore missed by American scientists. This has resulted in misinformation and a tenacious dependence on outdated theories that are not serving the American public.

When enzymes become your focus in food and health, you will be joining the ranks of those who are on the cutting edge of reaching their highest health potential.

MAKING THE CASE FOR ENZYME SUPPLEMENTS

The National Digestive Diseases Information Clearinghouse in Bethesda, Maryland, published these 1993 statistics for the United States as follows:

- 116,609 digestive system cancer deaths
- 20 million cases of gallstones
- 666 million reports of "heartburn" each month
- 20 million cases of irritable bowel syndrome
- 191,311 total deaths due to digestive diseases
- 22.3 million work-loss days due to acute indigestion
- 4.5 million hospitalizations due to indigestion
- 13 percent of total hospitalizations due to digestive disorders
- 5.8 million digestive system surgeries
- 7 percent of the total number of surgeries performed were digestive-system-related.[4]

---

[4]Victor P. Kulvinskas. *Don't Dine Without Enzymes.* Hot Springs, Ark.: L.O.V.E. Foods, Inc., 1994, p. 15.

▼

Medical doctors D.A. Lopez, R.M. Williams, and M. Miehlke, experts in enzyme therapy and research and authors of the book *Enzymes: The Fountain of Life*, tell us, "During the past 40 years, oral enzymes have been used in Europe and other countries as an approved, ethical and widely accepted modality of treatment for a variety of conditions."[5] They add that every year oral enzymes are used extensively outside the United States to treat millions of patients who suffer from arthritis, multiple sclerosis, autoimmune disorders, and cancer.

In referring to cancer, they write, "studies in Korea and Europe report an overall decrease in mortality and a decrease in relapse rates after oral therapeutic enzyme mixtures."[6]

Why are we not leading the world in this breakthrough technology? Drs. Lopez, Williams, and Miehlke explain: "The United States has lagged behind in enzyme research, primarily due to 'previous dogma' that minimizes their [enzymes] importance, and to confusion and contradiction in the American medical literature regarding their status.[7]

"Although not widely known in the United States or the Americas, the European research and experience has generated great excitement in the scientific community. The Europeans suggest that this knowledge can be used today to alleviate the pain which millions of people have had to suffer for years, and be used preventively to protect us from new illnesses and to provide us with a longer, healthier life."[8]

▲

The National Digestive Diseases Information Clearinghouse reports that *digestive disorders alone* cost 34 million Americans 200,000 absences from work each day (7.9 million annually) at a national cost of $50 billion a year, $17 billion of which are direct medical costs. Does that not greatly support the government urging for Americans to eat more fruits and vegetables? It

---

[5]D.A. Lopez, R.M. Williams, M. Miehlke. *Enzymes: The Fountain of Life*. Charleston, S.C.: Neville Press, Inc., 1994, p. 21.
[6]Ibid., p. 19.
[7]Ibid., p. 45.
[8]Ibid., p. 45.

would also make sense for enzyme supplements for digestion to be added to the recommended nutritional supplement charts.

Enzymes and Weight Loss

After taking enzyme supplements, we notice that our food doesn't sit in our stomachs, feeling like lead. Instead, within a short time after eating, we feel light, satisfied, and energetic.

When we began FITONICS workshops in 1993, many of our participants, after taking food enzymes for several weeks, reported an increased sense of well-being, as if, overall, their bodies were functioning more smoothly. Certainly, problems with elimination and constipation lessened for many. Everyone looked younger, brighter, more radiant and alive from eating more live food and taking enzyme supplements. Some reported that they were no longer taking the quantity of over-the-counter drugs they had been using.

One of our "superachievers," a charming Italian-American gentleman everyone called "Ralphie," became so passionate about enzyme supplements and enzyme-rich juices instead of the other heavy foods he loved that he lost thirty-six pounds in

---

**The Third Principle
of Natural Health and Weight Loss**

To improve digestion and get the most from food, we take enzyme supplements with every cooked food meal. Regular enzyme supplements can make a significant difference in our general health, well-being, and, consequently, in weight loss.

only ten weeks! Trudy, a sixty-five-year-old woman who had trouble walking, lost thirty-six pounds in four months and was out and about, energetically exercising. She landed a new job and her whole life changed!

Whether you notice immediate improvements in how you feel is not as important as the knowledge of the good you are doing by letting enzyme supplements perform the work of enhancing digestion. They contribute to your body's total health! Over the long term, you'll see such a dramatic

HOW TO USE ENZYME SUPPLEMENTS

Food enzyme supplements for aid in digestion are sold at General Nutrition Centers and natural food stores around the country. Look for a *full-spectrum* enzyme that contains *at least* protease, amylase, and lipase enzymes and take the recommended dosage with each cooked meal.

shift in appearance and well-being that you'll want all those you love to know about the importance of food enzymes.

Enzymes and Digestive Health

Indigestion is such a heartbreaking and unnecessary affliction. It results in so many widely experienced symptoms that no one should have to experience. High blood pressure, chest pain, heartburn, gas, nausea, a bloated feeling, belching, bad breath and body odors, headaches, stomach and abdominal pain, exhaustion, irritability, depression, sleeplessness, nightmares, cramping, constipation, diarrhea, irritable bowel syndrome, diverticulosis, food allergies, drug dependency, and mental impairments such as loss of memory and lack of concentration are all related to poor digestion. *The major cause of indigestion is the wide variety of enzyme-deficient cooked and processed foods Americans are eating.*

You may be wondering whether you need enzymes if you have no problem with digestion, or if you eat mostly live food.

Our bodies use up their enzymes in so many ways it pays to make deposits in your enzyme bank account regardless of what you eat. For example, enzymes are used up faster during illness, during extremely hot or cold weather, and during strenuous exercise. And since, from soil depletion and overprocessing, our food supply is devastatingly devitalized, you need all the energy you can muster to counteract that tragedy.

Always remember:

▶ Energy is the essence of your life.

▶ It takes enzymes to build energy.

▶ Food enzymes save your body's energy.

▶ Food that is efficiently digested can yield more energy for your body.

Enzymes and Longevity

We've already mentioned that, as you pass into your prime, the amount of enzymes your body can produce continues to decline and, as you have seen, low enzyme levels are associated with old age and chronic disease. But it doesn't have to be this way. As we have shown, evidence from research in Europe and Japan and from pioneering Natural Health specialists suggests that we have the ability to replenish our enzyme bank with enzyme supplements and conserve our enzymes by eating more live food, and perhaps extend our longevity.

What we are talking about is our very ability to lengthen the human life span, adding healthy, active, high-quality years to our lives. There is plenty of evidence to suggest that this is possible. Laboratory animals raised on live food live almost 30 percent longer than animals raised on cooked foods. If this holds true for human beings, it means you could extend your life by twenty (healthy) years or more!

The Japanese, who hold the lead position for longevity in the world, eat much of their fish and seafood raw. They cook their vegetables minimally and use large quantities of tamari or soy sauce, miso, and other condiments that are naturally fermented. This fermentation process in these foods creates active enzymes that work to predigest the food that is eaten with them.

Such soy products are probably the world's oldest enzyme agents, and they have been recognized in Asia for thousands of years for their digestion-promoting properties.[9] The Russian Abkhazians are among the longest-living people on earth, and main staples in their diets are fermented (enzyme-rich) raw sauerkraut and raw yogurt, which is full of enzymes as well.

Clearly, enzymes are a "found treasure." And they're not the only prize you will find on your quest for Natural Health. One of the great secrets of supermodels and superstars that you owe it to your own superself to understand is . . .

[9]Anthony J. Cichoke. *Enzymes and Enzyme Therapy*. New Canaan, Conn.: Keats Publishing, 1994, pp. 43–44.

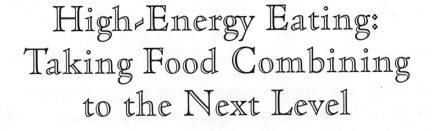

6

High-Energy Eating: Taking Food Combining to the Next Level

▼

*"Should you find yourself attending
a fashionable London dinner party
with Princess Diana,
don't offer her caviar on a cracker.
The princess, along with a clutch of other royals
(including, say rumormongers, Fergie),
rock stars and assorted celebs,
plus scads of everyday Brits,
has caught Hay fever—
a system of healthy eating
(developed just after the turn of the century
by an American physician, William Howard Hay)
that discourages, among other things,
dining on protein and starch at the same meal."*
—ANDREW WILSON,
"The Diet That Works for Di"
Fitness, January–February 1996

How to Be Supersexy!

Supermodels: Karen Alexander and Claudia Schiffer. Platinum recording stars: Reba McIntire and Cher. Television celebrities: Suzanne Somers, Mary Hart, and Candice Bergen. Hollywood hot properties: Woody Harrelson, Gene Hackman, and Ted Danson.

What do all these supersexy, high-energy achievers have in common? At some time or another, they have all avowed their enthusiasm for FIT FOR LIFE and the food-combining program it espoused.

If you never read *FIT FOR LIFE*, you are perhaps unaware that food combining is a formula for High Energy Eating that has been delineated in the works of many Natural Health pioneers, such as Dr. William Howard Hay, Dr. N.W. Walker, and Dr. Herbert Shelton. If you *have* read *FIT FOR LIFE*, you may be aware of the brouhaha over food combining the book created.

In effect, FIT FOR LIFE succeeded, for the first time in our history, in bringing food combining, developed over sixty years ago in this country as a breakthrough—a cost-free approach to healthful weight loss, energy, and disease prevention—to mainstream America and the world.

As you seek weight loss and a higher level of health, food combining is a handy *tool* to have at your disposal. In a nutshell, it's High Energy Eating, a simple, natural system that ensures a trim body, prevents constipation and indigestion, and gives you the kind of radiance and confidence about your health that keeps you supersexy.

Bah, Humbug?

Charles Darwin, the father of the Theory of Evolution, was also well known for his work as a taxonomist.[1] One day, wanting to test their professor, his students decided to play a trick on him. They combined the body parts of several insects into one. When they showed this "new" species to Darwin, he coined a word for it. Few of us realize that we can thank Darwin not only for the Theory of Evolution, but also for the popular term "humbug."

---

[1] A scientist who is a specialist in classifying plants and animals according to their presumed natural relationships.

As millions of *FIT FOR LIFE* readers were praising its effectiveness with dramatic and heartwarming testimonials, hundreds of thousands of letters flooded the FIT FOR LIFE offices:

"I've thrown away my antacids!"

"I've lost so much weight, but I never feel deprived."

"The arthritis in my knees is gone. Yesterday, I climbed a ladder and repaired my roof."

"I can't believe it! I'm no longer constipated!"

"I'm 89. I had such bad arthritis that I couldn't hold a pen. This letter I'm writing to you is the first I've written in years."

"My headaches are gone!"

"I was a size 12; now I'm down to an 8. My husband says I'm even sexier than when we were dating in high school."

Readers were dropping pounds like leaves from the trees in autumn, and they were feeling the boundless energy that is one of the side-benefits of food combining. Many were ending nearly **lifelong** dependence on antacids and laxatives. Chiropractors, massage therapists, homeopaths, and naturopathic physicians, as well as many forward-thinking nutritionists, dentists, dietitians, and medical doctors were openly excited about the positive effects of food combining on their patients' health and energy. They all began recommending *FIT FOR LIFE* to their patients.

But, Doctor, Have You Ever Tried It?

There is a great difference between an actual experience of truth and learned opinion. Although most medical doctors who have never studied food combining will tell you it doesn't matter what combinations you eat, in this chapter we will be revisiting the theory of food combining, one of the major Natural Health secrets to gaining energy and losing weight.

Just as American medical science has resisted research on food enzymes for health, it has equally ignored the potential value of this high-enzyme, disease-preventing, weight-loss tool. When we mentioned to a cardiologist friend of ours that information such as food combining could lower the number of patients who were seeking his help for wrong eating habits, his immediate comment was "Oh, we don't want to do that!" Do we? Heart disease is our runaway national killer, taking one out of two lives. Was our doctor friend exemplifying the unfortunate attitude that the *health* of the patient is less important than the *wealth* of the practitioner?

FOOD COMBINING GIVES US MORE ENERGY! From energy comes weight loss and good health. This is why we believe it is so relevant to your life and why we are redefining it for you in FITONICS. And we hope you get excited about it too!

As you systematically simplify your meals through this principle, you streamline digestion to prevent or eliminate constipation. The abundance of energy you save conserves enzymes. You may hear arguments for or against food combining, with all manner of sophisticated scientific rationales, but the bottom line is: *The application brings results!*

As we redefine this tool, we ask you to remember Charles Darwin. To argue against something that works and brings good to people's lives is "Humbug!"

Do you want more energy? Do you want to lose a few extra pounds? Do you want to throw out your antacids and laxatives? Do you want that svelte, supersexy feeling that comes from knowing you're taking care of your health? Then try food combining! Millions can testify to its effectiveness. And if you are not one of them, this is your chance to learn about it and make it a valuable tool in your life.

Again:
It Takes Energy
to Lose Weight

We cannot underscore this point often enough. *Successful weight loss depends on having an abundance of energy.* We've said repeatedly that energy is the ultimate commodity because we want you to take seriously the methods we are offering to help you conserve and build it. Food combining is one of those methods, and that's why we call it High Energy Eating.

FIT FOR LIFE repeatedly emphasized: The digestion of food demands more energy than any other bodily function. After what you've read so far, we're sure you won't argue with that. In fact, you also know this! Not only does digestion take more energy than anything else you attempt to do, but since you eat three times a day (at least) every day of your life, imagine how many of your enzymes it uses! A hefty percentage over the course of your lifetime! We hope that, by now, you're interested in any measure that will help you change that equation. If you still have doubts, let us help you connect to your experience of the toll on your energy that digestion takes.

What happens when you eat a large meal? Don't you get sleepy? That's because your body has shifted much of its energy requirement to digestion. It wants you to take a nap, since it has less energy for other vital processes. If you lie down, close your eyes, and remain still for a while, that will free up the energy it needs to break down all the food sitting in your stomach. Although a walk after a reasonable amount of food is healthier, a nap is what frequently happens when people overeat.

Think about Thanksgiving dinner. It's one of the best examples of what we're talking about. After leaving the holiday dinner table feeling absolutely stuffed, all you want to do is relax in the living room and wait until you feel there's a little room to squeeze in just one more small piece of pumpkin pie.

Think about how you feel after one of those long business lunches or dates with your friends when you end up eating more than you planned. Aren't you ready for a nap? Or a second cup of coffee?

A Tool, *Not* a Rule

Food combining is a tool you can use to stay healthy, the same kind of tool as, say, aerobic exercise. It's *not* a rule that you must obey at all costs, all the time, and feel like a failure if you break it. It's like a shirt you can take on and off; it's not a *straitjacket.* It's a tried-and-proven formula that will help you structure your eating to avoid constipation, weight gain, and stomach pain. It's a guideline that simplifies your digestive process. Simplifying, we repeat, will ensure that your body will have to expend less energy, which will result, as well, in enzyme conservation.

Now, how can that be bad? It is, in fact, the biggest benefit you will receive from food combining.

The Food Combining Process

If you look for research on food combining, the name of the famous Russian scientist Ivan Pavlov will "ring a bell." Known as well as the father of classical conditioning, in his studies on dogs, reported in *The Work of the Digestive Glands*, Pavlov discovered that meat and starch have different transit times in the stomach. He found that starch such as bread, potatoes, or pasta leaves the stomach in less than half the time of meat, which requires about four hours.

Pavlov was astounded, however, when he discovered that a mixed meal of meat and starch in his subjects took eight or more hours to leave the stomach! This means that traditional American sandwiches of meat and bread—the hamburger, hot dog, roast beef on a bun, ham and cheese or turkey on rye, to say nothing of all the meat and potatoes we eat—ALL take twice as long to leave our stomachs than the separate ingredients would if we ate the meat as a main course at one meal and the bread and/or potatoes as a main course at the next. Twice as long can mean twice the drain on your energy and enzymes.

In 1931, Dr. Lionel Picton, the chief author of the progressive *Cheshire Medical Testament* (in which thirty-one medical doctors espousing principles of Natural Health concurred that the prevention of sickness depends on correct feeding), maintained that a delay in the stomach means a delay throughout the entire digestive tract, which includes the colon: "The somewhat startling conclusion flows from this, that meals of mixed character, such as meat and bread, *favor* constipation, whereas meat and salad at one meal and starchy food such as bread and butter[2] at a separate meal have no such effect."[3]

The foremost pioneer in food combining was an American medical doctor, William Howard Hay, born in Hartstown, Pennsylvania, in 1866. Dr. Hay graduated from the University of New York in 1891, and during the next sixteen years he practiced medicine in the same manner as the rest of his medical colleagues. In his early forties, Dr. Hay's health began to decline, and he admitted that "he knew as little as the rest [of those in his profession] of the predisposing causes of disease."[4] As his condition worsened, Hay developed Bright's disease, high blood pressure, and an enlarged heart. Medical diagnosis by his colleagues was that he had only a short time to live.

But instead of giving in to disease, Dr. Hay turned toward the field of Natural Health. He ate, as he put it, "fundamentally" and "only such things as he believed were intended by Nature as food for man, taking them in natural form, and in quantities no greater than seemed necessary for his present need."[5]

---

[2]Author's note: Bread and butter with soup or vegetables.
[3]Doris Grant and Jean Joice. *Food Combining for Health*. Rochester, Vt.: Healing Arts Press, 1989, p. 40.
[4]Ibid., p. 17.
[5]Ibid., p. 17.

In following the principles of Natural Health, Hay overcame his illness. Within three months his symptoms were gone. He had lost fifty pounds, and he felt more fit than ever before. He turned toward the idea of treating disease through diet, a medically unorthodox approach for that (and this) era. He let it be known that "medicine was on the wrong track . . . fussing with the end results of a condition instead of attempting to remove the cause, for here was his own case recovering from a condition that the best authorities said was incurable."[6]

As the years passed and Hay became increasingly stronger and more willing to treat disease by his "surefire" natural methods, he faced the growing enmity of his colleagues with courage. He proved repeatedly in the treatment of his patients that "the body is merely a composite of what goes into it daily in the form of food and drink."[7]

In developing the system for which he became renowned, Hay always asserted that he had not invented anything new, but rather had learned to *remove the obstacles in the path of Nature's healing forces.*

The damaging acid that forms in the body as a result of incompatible food combinations was Dr. Hay's main focus. This acid reaction is so commonplace that billions of dollars are spent annually to advertise antacids to you, the unfortunate consumer, that will combat it. Rarely, however, do these ads even come close to telling you what a simple process it is to prevent acidity in the first place.

How to Prevent Acid Indigestion

When proteins—such as meat, poultry, fish, eggs, and dairy— and carbohydrates—such as bread, rice, potatoes, or pasta—are eaten at the same meal, as is routinely done at practically every

[6]Ibid., p. 18.
[7]Ibid., p. 18.

meal eaten in this country, the inefficient digestion that results causes serious acidity. To grasp this concept, a basic understanding of simple chemistry is required. Proteins in the body break down in hydrochloric acid. Starches require the alkalinity of ptyalin in the saliva for their initial digestion. When ample quantities of proteins and starches are eaten simultaneously, the effectiveness of the alkaline and acid digestive juices is seriously diminished. There is too much acid to permit the starch to be digested, but not enough acid to digest the protein.

In effect, ptyalin and hydrochloric acid have partially neutralized each other. When protein is incompletely digested, it putrefies. Incompletely digested starches ferment. Fats in the same predicament turn rancid. And with what we've learned in the last chapters about the importance of enzymes to digestion and our enzyme-deficient diet of cooked foods, most of our mixed meals of proteins and starches are in all likelihood beginning to spoil in the cardiac stomach, because there are no enzymes to predigest them!

All of these unhealthful situations result in acid in your body. In the next chapter, you will learn exactly why, from this point on, you will wish to prevent acidity as often as you can.

Dr. Hay published the first book on the subject of food combining in the 1930s. Decades ahead of its time, the book focused on the acid effect and the hidden cost to vitality of incompatible mixtures of foods that were routinely being eaten. He talked about combinations to help us receive the most benefit from the fruit we are eating. He clarified how to have dessert healthfully. And specifically, he warned that as we continually eat chemically incompatible combinations, such as proteins and starches at the same meal, we build up a tolerance to the ill effects that mask the harm they are causing, just as we can build an unnatural tolerance to drugs or coffee (we have to take more and more over time to get the same effect).

After decades of research, William Howard Hay gave us a most valuable guideline for prevention of ill health—*that starches should not be eaten with proteins at the same meal.* Practically speaking, this means Dr. Hay felt it was best to avoid such traditional combinations as bread and meat, chicken and noodles, or fish and rice, whenever possible. Hay found that if we reorganize our meals to feature either protein or starch, each combined with plenty of vegetables (and not with each other), we can be healthier and not suffer from a weight problem.

Typical questions that immediately come up are:

"Does that mean I can have two proteins together, like some shrimp and then chicken, as long as I eat lots of vegetables and salad with them?" Or,

"Can I have two starches together, like pasta and bread, as long as I add lots of vegetables?"

The answer to both is "YES." You can have a "hearty" steak with cheese on your salad. You can have mashed potatoes and whole grain bread—as long as you are also eating plenty of vegetables at the same meal.

Beans, Beans, the "Musical" Fruit

This one aspect of the theory of food combining, recommending the separation of proteins and starches (our meat-and-potato habit), was attacked vociferously by spokespeople for traditional medicine from the American Medical Association and the American Dietetic Association when it was first introduced in FIT FOR LIFE. Critics with the most orthodox credentials argued that Nature herself combines proteins and starches in most foods, so if proteins and starches are an incompatible mixture, then Nature has made a mistake.

Of course, we all know that Nature combines proteins and starches in most foods, but we also understand that one of those almost always predominates. Sure there's some protein in bread or rice, but in far less significant quantities than the starch or carbohydrate content. And the *only* protein that contains any *significant* carbohydrates is dairy.

The food combining theory concerns *concentrated* proteins that are 20 percent or more protein. These are the animal proteins such as poultry, meat, fish, cheese, and milk. Similarly, in referring to starches, it is always *concentrated* starches, which are 20 percent or more carbohydrate, that are being considered. These are cereals, grains, potatoes, and refined sugars.

There is only *one* food in Nature that contains relatively equal amounts of protein and carbohydrates, and, if anything, it disperses the "hot air" of the critics and thoroughly *proves* the food combining principle. This is the legume family—dried peas, beans, lentils, and peanuts. What happens when you eat these foods? In all likelihood, you experience gas, bloating, and discomfort—sometimes painful (and sometimes embarrassingly audible) **feedback** confirming the food combining theory that proteins and starches are incompatible in the digestive tract.

Food Combining, the FITONICS Way— No Fanaticism, Please

The research Dr. Hay initiated on food combining spawned a variety of expressions of the theory in the sixty years or more during which it has been in use. Although the protein/starch guideline remains constant, we have uncovered ways to make the use of it as practical and effective as possible.

When you are monitoring your protein/starch combinations, focus on the *main items* on your plate, not on a sprinkling of Parmesan cheese on your pasta or salad. We're frequently asked:

"What if there's a little chicken in my soup?"

"What if there's a little yogurt in my salad dressing? Does that mean I can't have any carbs?"

"Can I have milk on my cereal?"

Our answer: Avoid being fanatic about this theory. Remember, it is a *tool* to lose weight and increase energy, not a rule that can never be broken. Use it when it's relevant. A little cheese on pasta or a few bits of turkey or ham in your soup are not what we are talking about. Please understand, all conceptions of amounts of food are relative. In other words, we're talking about small amounts . . . not a shovelful.

---

*Food combining applies
to the main items on your plate,
not to the traces or condiments.*

You can use cheese or yogurt in *small* quantities with rice or other starches; you can add an ounce of chicken to your pasta, or fish to your rice, as long as the amounts remain negligible and *vegetables predominate.* Conversely, you may be having grilled chicken with salad and, lo and behold, there are some croutons on the salad. You can pick them out or eat them. A few croutons are not going to make a significant difference.

As for milk on cereal, we have found a palate-pleasing solution. We often substitute soy milk (plain or vanilla flavored) for dairy milk, because soy milk is lower in protein and higher in carbs than dairy milk. As such, it is more compatible than dairy milk with cereals.

If you look to the Asians and the East Indians, whose traditional protein has for centuries been far less than that in Western society, you will notice that they routinely mix small quantities of protein with starches and vegetables. The Chinese balance their rice dishes with slivers of pork or chicken. The Japanese balance their bowls of noodles with *vegetables* and bits of dried fish. The Hindus add dairy healthfully to grains and legumes, in very *small* quantities, overwhelmed by vegetables. In all of these cultures, the proteins are in lesser amounts than the typical American "quarter- or half-pounder."

Our problem stems from our tendency to sit down to a 16-ounce steak or half a roast chicken with a large serving of potatoes, several slices of bread—and a token salad or vegetable, off to the side, as if it were a garnish. Food combining is most relevant when you are looking at the main portions of foods, not garnishes. And since it leads us to turn to vegetables and salads as the sole accompaniment to our protein or starch entrees, it's a surefire way to bring more health-building, slenderizing raw and cooked vegetables into our lives.

The Power Lunch and the Soothing Supper

If you are a meat eater seeking High Energy from your meals while losing weight and avoiding acidity and the constipation that frequently accompany meat eating, we have found that meats are digested most efficiently when they're eaten with salads and vegetables.

This is our recommended POWER LUNCH. We give it this name because proteins actually *stimulate* and bring about clear thinking. Eaten with enzyme-rich salads and high-fiber vegetables, they create the perfect mental energy for getting your work accomplished in the afternoon.

On the other hand, carbohydrates cause your brain to secrete serotonin, which makes you sleepy. For this reason, we recommend the SOOTHING SUPPER when you can focus on starches, which go down smoothly when they are combined with cooked vegetables.

In other words, eat one type of meal at lunch and the other at dinner, and your life will become easier. For example, an ideal lunch would be a large mixed salad with egg salad; a chef's salad with meats; a Caesar salad with grilled chicken. On a cold day, you could add a bowl of vegetable soup or hot herbal tea. An ideal dinner would be rice and vegetables; soup and thick slices of hot, whole-grain bread; or mashed potatoes, gravy, and vegetables.

We have also found that dairy with starches is a far less burdensome combination than meat with starches. The most ancient vegetarian cuisine has *always* incorporated dairy. So you *can* have an occasional pizza! Especially if it's one of those wonderful grilled or roasted vegetable pizzas, and especially after you've dropped 30 pounds and are on to maintenance. Asking for *extra* vegetables and lighter cheese is one of the secrets to keeping the weight off.

For vegetarians who enjoy tofu as their principle protein source, unless they are truly low on energy or have lots of weight to lose, combining tofu, an enzymatically predigested protein, with starches poses no obstacles. And immediately another question comes up:

"Does that mean I can never have a hamburger on a bun, never have mashed potatoes with my turkey?"

REMEMBER, THIS IS A *TOOL*! NOT A *RULE*! Don't make it a dietary death sentence! It's most useful and important for weight loss or when you are low on energy. Of course you're going to fully celebrate Thanksgiving with friends and family. *We do!* And you can have a hamburger on a bun occasionally (or maybe you'll opt for the veggieburger on the whole-wheat bun). In either case, pile it high with lettuce, tomatoes, and sprouts, for the enzymes. You can have meatballs and spaghetti! With a big salad! We could go on and on and on . . . giving you permission that we are asking you to give yourself, *whenever appropriate.*

**The Fourth Principle
of Natural Health and Weight Loss**

To lose weight and increase energy,
avoid routinely mixing proteins and starches.
Have proteins with salads and nonstarchy
vegetables at lunch (the Power Lunch)
and starches with vegetables and/or salads
at dinner (the Soothing Supper).

You know what you need, and you know how you want to play this game to feel most comfortable. There's no "food cop" in your life anymore. YOU'RE IN CHARGE! When you come to the crossroads and make the choice to follow the path to Natural Health, the pace is up to you. Just remember, the days when you *do* monitor your combinations of foods will be the days when you drop an extra pound, build a little more energy, and feel a little sexier!

Speaking of Sex, What About Desserts?

We get as many questions about sex as about dessert, so we'll put the first question "to bed" first. Sex requires an abundance of energy for peak performance! If you want better sex, then don't waste all your energy on digestion. It also helps not to be constipated. Food combining delivers in both these areas. Now back to desserts.

Dr. Hay gave us a guideline. Since desserts are usually of a starchy nature, **they should be eaten *only* if your main course** consists of starches and vegetables—*not* after a Power Lunch, but after the Soothing Supper. In other words, they are perfectly compatible with a vegetarian (starch-and-vegetable) meal. **Desserts of a starchy nature are *incompatible* when you have eaten a protein entree.**

It's common sense if you are not going to routinely mix proteins and carbohydrates as you set your sights on slenderizing and energizing, you aren't going to mix proteins with desserts that are also carbohydrates. Therefore, you can have dessert if you have had a simple meal such as rice and vegetables. One of our favorite meals at the end of the day is hot vegetable soup and whole-grain bread followed by a thick slice of sweet potato pie.

How to Benefit from Enzyme-Rich Fruit

FIT FOR LIFE made a very big deal over fruit. The book recommended that fruit *only* be eaten alone, on an empty stomach, and *never* be eaten with any other food. The explanation for this principle that so many have used successfully for so long was that *since fruit is 90 to 95 percent water, it will give your body an "inner bath" when eaten by itself.* Eaten on top of other foods, the theory is impeded in its tendency to "wash" through the digestive tract. For this reason, the fruit meal in the morning was emphasized as the very best time for eating fruit, when the stomach is empty.

It is time to update the fruit principle. Fruit is one of the best donors of enzymes to our bodies that we can find. We have discovered several ways over the course of the decade since *FIT FOR LIFE* was written to increase our opportunities to eat fruit throughout the day, while taking advantage of the enzymes it contains to expedite the digestion of other heavier foods. Much of what follows is based on our direct experience and data from Dr. Hay's work.

▶ First and foremost, fruit combines *very* well with raw vegetables. A fruit salad can contain avocado and be accompanied by a large mixed vegetable salad, with a nonoily, dairy-based dressing. It is very important, especially during the warmer weather when you are eating live food, to understand how valuable fruit and vegetable meals can be.

▶ Second, certain fruits actually *facilitate* the digestion of proteins and others do the same for starches. This flies in the face of the food combining guideline of FIT FOR LIFE, but let's face it, either we streamline our knowledge of nutrition over a decade or we stay stuck, holding on to an idea that may not be as cutting-edge as we would like it to be. We now have a better understanding of the value of enzymes as they work in the Food Enzyme (cardiac) stomach. We want to give the cooked foods we eat the *most* enzyme support we can from the live foods we eat with them.

After exploring Dr. Hay's work in depth, we agree that the addition of fruit to *compatibly combined* POWER LUNCHES or SOOTHING SUPPERS is a viable option.

Fruits That Help Digest Proteins

apples	nectarines	sour plums
apricots	oranges	raspberries
blueberries	papayas	strawberries
grapefruit	peaches	tangerines
kiwi	pears	
lemons	pineapples	

Fruits That Help Digest Starches

bananas	papayas
dates	very sweet pears
fresh and dried figs	very sweet plums
sweet grapes	raisins
mango	

An obvious example of using fruit to help digest a protein meal would be: chicken, a salad with a lemon juice-based dressing and some fresh sliced pineapple, kiwi, and orange. New World Cuisine, introduced in the cutting-edge restaurants in Miami, Florida, and now influencing gourmet chefs around the country, skillfully mixes fruit with protein by topping fresh grilled fish with fresh fruit salsas. Another classic protein-fruit combination is a fruit salad topped with yogurt, or fruit and cheese. For a change of pace, we enjoy adding sliced strawberries, oranges, or raspberries to a green salad, instead of tomatoes when we are eating salad with protein. As a dessert, when you are eating a protein and vegetables, you may delight in a bowl of fresh strawberries with a little yogurt. Skip the sponge cake with all its sugar!

An obvious and commonplace example of mixing fruit with starches for better digestion would be the addition of sliced banana and raisins to a high-fiber cereal, topping it, for added enjoyment, with soy milk, or the addition of pears to oatmeal. Raisins or currants added to rice or couscous is also digestively helpful.

One of our favorite ways to enjoy fruit with starch is the updated peanut butter sandwich. We use a whole, multigrain bread, toasted lightly and spread with almond butter, sliced banana, and lots of alfalfa sprouts. No matter what we eat, we try to add sprouts whenever they're tastefully relevant, since they are *sprouting, still growing*, and therefore, so bursting with life— enzymes!

There's a certain amount of common sense here. You will notice from the above lists that juicier fruits seem to work best with proteins, while the very surgery, starchy fruits complement starches.

Perhaps by now you've noticed that vegetables are neutral. They go with *everything*. If you wanted carrot juice or even to eat a carrot with cereal, that would be great! The more enzymes the better.

In all of the above examples of healthful fruit consumption, you are not only increasing your enzyme intake, but you are also making your meals more exciting and enjoyable, which goes a long way to making these tools part of your lifestyle.

One Caveat

If you are mixing fruits with other foods, be sure that you eat them *with* the foods or *immediately* after, so they can mix together in the Food Enzyme stomach where predigestion takes place. The enzymatic nature of the fruits will actually facilitate the digestion of proteins or starches in the Food Enzyme (cardiac) portion of the stomach. If you wait an hour or two after a cooked meal to eat fruit, and the food has passed into the lower part of the stomach, you risk indigestion. When fruit comes into contact with food in a more advanced state of digestion, it interferes with the digestive process. We have found from practical experience that fruit between meals interferes with the work of the digestive acids in the lower portion of the stomach.

In other words, unless you enjoy indigestion and the accompanying ill health and weight gain that can result, remember Pavlov! He told us that meat takes four hours to leave the stomach while starch takes two and a half hours. According to his research, meat and starch eaten together can be in the stomach eight hours or longer! So . . . after your POWER LUNCH of protein and vegetables, wait four hours before having a helpful and healthful enzyme-rich fruit snack. Wait two and a half hours after a SOOTHING SUPPER or other starch-based meal. If you eat meat and starch together, you probably won't want fruit for eight hours or more. So if you have an occasional breakfast or brunch of Eggs Benedict, the perfect supper, at least eight hours later, will be your missed fruit meal from the morning! See how it works? It's a game worth playing!

Mom and Apple Pie

FIT FOR LIFE admonished against the cooking of any fruit, warning that cooked fruit adds acidity to the body. This was a guideline from the field of Natural Health developed as an alternative to medicines and surgery for healing of the seriously ill. Natural Health has developed a tendency over the years to advocate a rather stringent raw food diet, which has been a remarkably successful therapy for many people. Coming from a broader base, with ten additional years to experiment on the most *practical* eating lifestyle, in FITONICS we take a different position to the one *FIT FOR LIFE* advocated on cooked fruit. In a nutshell, *FIT FOR LIFE* put cooked fruit off limits.

Although enzyme-rich fresh fruit is one of the most valuable foods you can eat, along with fresh vegetables, cooked fruit is still a viable food choice. Certainly, broiled pineapple and grapefruit, a baked apple, or poached pears is less harmful than the negative elements of high-fat meats, coffee, or sugar. Cooked fruit adds warmth and variety to your menus, and a good dose of fiber.

Since you lose the enzymes when the fruit is cooked, we always make sure to replenish them with food enzyme supplements, and we eat plenty of fresh vegetables at the same meal. For example, a large mixed vegetable salad with a Banana-Date Bread Pudding or a baked apple would be an excellent way to have cooked fruit. This is healthful and homey "sweet eating," and it creates an atmosphere of love and nourishment in a happy home. It's always better to err on the side of a whole-grain bread pudding or a baked apple than a candy bar.

Change Is Good!

For those who have diligently followed the *FIT FOR LIFE* guidelines on fruit and the recommendation that it never be combined with any other food, these new suggestions are coming at a time when you may be ready for some change. TRY THEM! You may see, as we have over the years, that more liberal guidelines regarding fruit do make the eating experience more pleasurable. They also assist rather than thwart digestion.

Not a Panacea, but They *Will* Help

We find that taking digestive enzymes mitigates the drop in energy and retarded digestion that result when we choose to ignore food combining. With enzyme supplements, predigestion in the Food Enzyme, or cardiac, stomach works to offset the digestive problems that incompatible combinations produce.

However, notwithstanding the benefit of digestive enzymes, we don't routinely ask our bodies to do more than they can do easily. Why burden them? It's we who pay the price! If you have to walk five miles, do you do it carrying a backpack full of weights? Not if you have a choice! If putting proteins and starches into your stomach at the same meal drains your precious energy, why not learn the trick of eating so that doesn't happen. At least, not all the time! We find ourselves compatibly combining proteins and starches in approximately 70 percent of our meals.

What You Can Expect to Hear . . .

Here are some of the arguments against food combining that will inevitably come up as you begin to notice that, when you use it, you lose weight and gain energy.

"Humbug," some doctors and/or dietitians may say. "Your stomach can handle *any* combination of foods, just like the stomach of a rat. You're an omnivore."

When you hear that official-sounding brush-off, remember that although our stomachs may be able to *handle* any combination of foods, there is a price we pay. Consider the ancient Hebrew principle that "the body is the temple of the indwelling spirit." If we think of our bodies as temples, we will treat them with profound respect, maintaining them in the ways that keep us most healthy and whole.

Thus, when food combining is attacked, our answer is: Please ask yourself if it works for *you*. If food combining benefits you, if you feel better, does it matter to you if some representatives of traditional medicine—most of whom spend less than 12 hours of their training in nutrition or are focused on symptom fighting instead of prevention—say it doesn't make sense to them? If food combining works for you, *use it!* It is one of the best natural ways for building health and preventing ill health.

Skeptics Say Our Stomachs Can Handle Anything: But Look at the Facts

Dr. Hay's work on food combining and the success of *FIT FOR LIFE* exemplify results in people's lives. In spite of bitter attacks from his medical colleagues for his theory, he was able to restore normal health to countless people whose cases had been termed "hopeless" by medical authorities. His work was far ahead of its time, as his detractors maintained that food and nutrition played no relevant role in health.

Today we know differently, and if Hay were here now, using his principles in practice, we believe he'd be conveying a message millions would want to hear. But in his own lifetime, in this country, Hay's concepts were rejected with scorn, and he was constantly subjected to the vehement opposition of entrenched medical orthodoxy.[8] (Despite its massive success, *FIT FOR LIFE*, as well, underwent unrelenting attacks from the American Medical Association and the American Dietetic Association because of this one principle.)

▼

We have a $5 billion market for heartburn (indigestion) medications in this country.[9] There's an industry war over profits from such over-the-counter standbys as Tums, Rolaids, Maalox, Mylanta, and the prescription drugs Zantac, Tagamet, Pepcid, and Axid, which went over the counter in November 1995 to a hail of fanfare. Indigestion, as we have earlier pointed out, is a veritable industry in our country. Don't you think that fact might indicate that our stomachs *can't* handle everything we're told they can?

Studies revealed in October 1995 show that antacids and the new over-the-counter drugs such as Tagamet may mask symptoms of bleeding ulcers among people with rheumatoid arthritis. They also tell us that Tums and Rolaids can contribute to kidney stones, and that Mylanta and Maalox can be dangerous for those with kidney problems.[10]

Millions of people have first-stage kidney problems—and most of them don't even know it. Fighting symptoms rather than focusing on prevention is just like setting a fire in the middle of your living room and saying that it doesn't matter because there's a fire department in town. Why set the fire in the first place? Why eat to cause pain, weight gain, and low energy if you don't have to?

▲

It should not surprise you, however, that Dr. Hay was well received in other countries—particularly in England, where more enlightened medical doctors use food combining to this day to achieve results that cannot be attained by other methods. And *FIT FOR LIFE*, as well, sold more copies per capita in such advanced countries as Sweden, Germany, Israel, and Australia than the millions it sold in the United States.

---

[8]Grant and Joice. *Food Combining for Health*, p. 21.
[9]*Time*, November 6, 1995, p. 58.
[10]Ibid., p. 58.

Seeing Is Believing

If you're looking for proof that the theory of food combining holds true for all of the people all of the time, we'd like to ask you if you can find documentation that the taking of aspirin or any of the thousands of other pharmaceuticals is good for all the people all the time.

But still, one could argue: "I've eaten hamburgers and fish sandwiches in the past and I've felt just fine! I've had pizza with cheese on it with no adverse reaction!" Of course you have! Your body adjusts to whatever you do routinely. But no doubt there are times when you've felt your energy plummet. Your stomach has hurt. You've been constipated the next day.

The fact is: The energy you've wasted won't necessarily be experienced as immediate pain. It will be cumulative, contributing to weight gain, constipation, and general breakdowns in your body such as colds, headaches, sore muscles, hair loss, wrinkles, poor eyesight or hearing, and other more serious maladies. The bottom line is energy—and whether you are wasting it or conserving it. Whatever you do that throws your body out of balance is wasting your energy.

All we can ask is that you *try* food combining as your key to High Energy Eating. Once you do, like us and so many millions of *FIT FOR LIFE* enthusiasts, you'll realize that *food combining leaves you feeling more energetic.*

If you suffer from a weight problem, indigestion, constipation, or low energy, try food combining. It's something we know you'll be able to take to the bank . . . your enzyme bank! Have a fruit tonic, a POWER LUNCH, or a SOOTHING SUPPER, whatever the case may be. Begin with your very next meal. You will soon be looking slim and trim, and feeling sexy, with bundles of energy to match—and you'll be allowing your body to take care of one of its most critical tasks as it maintains . . .

7

▼

Homeostasis: The Acid-Alkaline Game

▼

"Dr. Theodore A. Baroody, Jr.,
author of several health books and a person involved
in studying spiritual evolution,
has suggested, based on his own
personal and clinical experience,
that as one evolves spiritually,
the body becomes lighter and transforms
physiologically to become more alkaline."

—GABRIEL COUSENS, *CONSCIOUS EATING*

"Homeostasis" is a term that refers to the tendency of your body to maintain its equilibrium by balancing its chemistry. Specifically, the most important equilibrium it must maintain is the condition of your blood. Authorities agree that if you wish to be healthy, your blood must be alkaline, rather than acid.

The actual healthy pH of the blood falls within a narrow range of between 7.35 and 7.45. Experts also agree that values above or below this range create drastic, potentially fatal, consequences.

For example, Dr. Paavo Airola, Natural Health pioneer and world-famous nutritionist, believed that acidosis (an acidic bloodstream) is the basic cause of all disease. He also believed that when there is an excess of acids in the body, the body will maintain its balance (homeostasis) by depositing those acids in the tissues and joints, therefore contributing to the onset of arthritis.

If you are acidic, your body will give you plenty of clues. In *The Miracle of Fasting*, Dr. Paul Bragg writes: "From headache and indigestion, to pimples and common cold, most of our miseries arise from acidosis. The signs are many . . . dizziness, specks in the vision, bitterness in the mouth, physical slackness, and mental blockage . . . a grayish tongue, a snappish temper, a flushing of the face."[1]

We have found that one of the first signs to look for is dark circles under the eyes. But in essence, when your body is too acidic, it's fighting an uphill battle. It will expend tremendous energy working toward the alkaline balance. What an unfortunate scenario! That energy *could* be put toward the shedding of excess pounds.

One of the keys to Natural Health is an understanding that not only is your blood alkaline, but this holds true for all the other fluids and tissues of your body. One exception to this is your stomach, which has a special lining to handle its acid environment. When that protective lining breaks down from excess acidity, you get ulcers. A second exception is your urine, which will be alkaline or acid, reflecting how your body is at work to maintain homeostasis.

An Underlying Cause of Excess Weight

In addition to the theory of food combining, Dr. William Howard Hay taught his patients an additional point: that disease (and remember that excess weight is disease) has one underlying cause—an imbalanced chemistry and the loss of equilibrium (homeostasis) in the body. This situation is created by acidic end products of digestion and metabolism in far greater

---

[1]*The Miracle of Fasting.* Santa Barbara, Calif.: Health Science, 1992, pp. 30–31.

amounts than the body itself can eliminate. With thwarted elimination, Hay explained, we develop a condition of self-poisoning.[2] This results in acidity, a subsequent lowering of the body's alkaline reserves, and a dramatic decline in health.

In his research and treatment Hay accounted for five basic causes of acid imbalance.

Five Basic Causes of Acid Imbalance

1. Incompatible food combinations, principally the mixing of proteins and starches

2. Constipation

3. Overconsumption of meat

4. Overconsumption of refined carbohydrates, such as white flour and sugar

5. Inadequate intake of fruits and vegetables

Acid burns. This is common sense. Pour some on your hand and the results will be painful and ugly. Inside your body, acids can have the same effect over time. They age your tissues, cause your skin to wrinkle and wither, and create pain and bloating as your body wisely retains water to dilute them and keep them from literally destroying your organs.

The only exception to this, as we have said, is in your stomach, with its special lining to handle its acid environment. At some time or other, you have probably experienced a "gastric reflux," or regurgitation, when acid from your stomach bubbled into your esophagus and you felt the burning. So a certain amount of acid in the stomach is natural. But when your diet is

---

[2]Also called toxemia, metabolic imbalance, or auto-intoxication.

highly acid-forming, the stomach lining cannot withstand the excess, and you feel pain and experience acid indigestion.

Knowledge That Can Set You Free

Your body is a chemical laboratory that is continuously at work at the job of maintaining homeostasis. Knowing this will enable you to take greater control over your weight and your health. When your blood becomes too acidic, your body is forced to use its alkaline reserves—minerals such as calcium, potassium, sodium, iron, and magnesium—to neutralize the acid. When excess acidity causes a drain on your alkaline reserves, there is a weakening of your overall system. You're suffering from acidosis.

When the iron-rich hemoglobin in your blood is drained to neutralize the acids, fatigue sets in. When calcium, the mineral that keeps you calm and allows you to sleep, is drained, you're irritable and restless. Borrowing alkaline reserves from the nerves will have an effect on mental functioning and clarity. (Perhaps there is even a connection between alkaline deficiency and the epidemic of depression in our country.)

Common sense tells you that borrowing alkaline minerals from the bones will have a deleterious effect on your skeleton. We personally believe, as do many medical doctors and Natural Health pioneers, that when calcium is leached from the bones to neutralize acids, osteoporosis results. Since acidosis is so rampant, the daily intake of a plant-based mineral tonic will replace the minerals that are continuously being drained from the body.

Visualize for a moment the cells in your body. There is within each one of them an intricate alkaline environment dependent on an adequate supply of alkaline mineral salts. If your blood becomes even slightly acidic, the cells must sacrifice their minerals. At that moment, you have an acidic cell . . . in deep trouble.

Why? Enzyme function is suppressed in an acidic environment. Without active enzymes, intercellular activity begins to break down. From what you now know about enzymes, you can understand how serious that is. Your cells are your individual building blocks and you're only as strong and as healthy as your cells.

Many of the symptoms of acidosis are commonly experienced and misinterpreted. Fatigue and muscle stiffness, lower back pain, irritability, tension in the neck and shoulders, arthritis and osteoporosis, stomachaches, nausea, vomiting, chest pain, gastritis, ulcers, and constipation. Cancer cells thrive in an acidic environment while normal cells decline.

How to Avoid Alkaline Deficiency

Deep breathing calms and relaxes you. That's why it's used in meditation, Lamaze training, and for natural childbirth. That's why massage therapists may ask you to breathe deeply as they work on a sore muscle. **Deep breathing will balance your chemistry as it alkalinizes your blood by removing carbon dioxide from your body.**

Carbon dioxide is acidic. As you breathe deeply, you take in more oxygen and are forced to exhale more carbon dioxide. In addition to deep breathing, rest, optimistic thinking, fresh air, and exercise also help maintain homeostasis.

And it probably won't surprise you that the strongest influence on the condition of your blood is . . . you guessed it! Your diet! The foods you choose to eat will have an acidifying or alkalinizing effect.

Unfortunately, the Standard American Diet is decidedly acidifying. The meat, chicken, fish, pasteurized dairy, sodas, refined and whole grains, refined sugars, and junk foods that are its basis all acidify your bloodstream. Preservatives and most additives are acid-forming. So are alcohol, coffee, tea, drugs, candy, chocolate, cooked or unripe fruits, commercial vinegars, and tobacco. Peanuts, which are not nuts at all but legumes, and peanut butter are acid-forming. It seems that many of the items on this list come up repeatedly as we look for the causes of our problems.

Does this mean you have to give up all these foods and substances? No, but it would serve you well to learn a new equation about acid and alkaline foods. Knowing which foods help neutralize acids and using these foods in large enough quantities to control acidosis is an important key to Natural Health.

In doing so, you will find yourself focusing on the same foods that contain the enzymes you are seeking: Live (raw) vegetables and most live (raw) and ripe fruits, especially melons, are alkaline. Even the so-called acid fruits, such as citrus, pineapple, and tomatoes, eaten in their raw states, will have an alkaline effect in your body after digestion.

All fresh fruits and vegetable juices are alkaline, such as fresh carrot, watermelon, and green vegetable juices. If you're one of the many people with a juicer stored under your sink, it's time to pull it out and take advantage of what it can do for you. Or . . . become a regular patron at the excellent fresh juice stores opening all over this country as the Natural Health revolution gains momentum.

Also, sprouts, unpasteurized honey, herbal teas, raw almonds and almond butter, tofu, miso soup, sea vegetables, and algaes are also alkaline.

Supplemental, plant-based enzymes are alkaline, as well as the green algae and plant supernutrient powders we recommend you add to your morning tonics. Wheat grass juice, introduced by Natural Health pioneers Dr. Ann Wigmore and Victor Kulvinksas, is rich in alkalinity.

Since grains and legumes are such an important part of the Eating Right Pyramid guidelines for diet in our country, it is important to know how they fit into the acid/alkaline equation.

Two of the commonly eaten beans, limas and azukis, are alkaline. All other beans are acidic. With the exception of buckwheat and millet, all grains are acid as well. *However, all beans and grains become alkaline if they are soaked and sprouted and eaten raw in salads.*

This is a form of predigestion that also applies to nuts and seeds. Soaking removes the enzyme inhibitors that naturally coat all grains, seeds, nuts, and legumes. This is the same phenomenon that takes place when you are planting. It takes moisture for sprouting to occur, and no seed will ever grow without moisture. Once that sprouting process is set in motion, the end product will be alkaline. Soaking of grains, legumes, nuts, and seeds also converts fats to fatty acids, proteins to amino acids, and starches to sugars as enzyme activity is initiated. This predigestion lightens the digestive burden on your body.

To apply this information practically:

► Soak all raw nuts or seeds thirty minutes before eating them.

► Soak grains thirty minutes before cooking them. Pour off soaking water and cook in fresh water.

► Soak beans overnight before cooking them or use the fast soaking method: Boil for one minute and allow to stand, covered, for one hour. Pour off soaking water and cook in fresh water.

► Soak all seeds, grains, and legumes that you wish to sprout for at least an hour before draining and setting in a dark place for sprouting.

All foods have acid and alkaline properties. Whether the net effect will be acidifying or alkalinizing in your body is determined by which element predominates. Our ability to use this information in controlling our acid/alkaline balance gives us newfound control over our health.

Reorganize Your Diet

Dr. Hay felt that it was necessary to organize our diets to continuously replace our alkaline reserves. It is well known to physiologists that we need *four times* as much alkaline food in our diet as acid food to replace the losses that routinely occur. This means our diet should be approximately 75 percent alkaline food.

In *Back to Eden*, the classic guide to herbal medicine that was written in 1939 and is still in print, Jethro Kloss recommends: "75 to 85 percent alkaline foods should be used in the everyday diet. If you have any ailments, your diet should be at least 90 percent alkaline-forming foods."[3] The success of *FIT FOR LIFE* can be attributed to the 80 percent alkaline diet it encouraged.

FITONICS Prevents Acidosis

Please don't be overwhelmed by the percentages. This is much easier to maintain than you realize. *FIT FOR LIFE* taught us to eat a fresh fruit meal in the morning. FITONICS, utilizing the same principle, also encourages that morning fruit meal with the addition of the highly alkaline, green supernutrient tonic.

If that meal is quite sizable, we've already chalked up 30 percent of our daily intake of alkaline foods at the start of the day.

For those of you who didn't read *FIT FOR LIFE*, fruit in the morning facilitates the body's natural "elimination cycle," which is heightened from four A.M. to twelve noon every day. At that time of day your body has the most energy to rid itself of acids and excess weight.[4] If you forgo fruit and instead eat

---

[3]Jethro Kloss. *Back to Eden*. Loma Linda, Calif.: Eden Publishing, 1939, p. 7200.

[4]"To put it in its simplest terms, on a daily basis, we take in food (appropriation), we absorb and use some of that food (assimilation), and we get rid of what

acidic bacon and eggs or cereal, you thwart your body's attempt to maintain homeostasis by further acidifying your blood, and you put off weight loss.

For this reason, the "fruit in the morning" principle alone in *FIT FOR LIFE* produced such excellent results for readers that it created millions of "fruit in the morning" aficionados. Those who loved the principle did so because they felt and looked so much better using it.

Once you habituate yourself to that fresh, live, alkaline meal first thing in the morning, you will rarely want to break the habit. It's like your morning shower ritual, which cleans you every day on the outside. A fruit meal in the morning is your inner shower, helping to keep you clean, fresh, and young on the inside. That cleanliness radiates to the outside.

If you incorporate more salads and sprouts into your diet (for example, a large salad every day as part of your Power Lunch), your alkaline food intake will now be 45 percent. Try to include **many** raw vegetables and sprouts in your salads along with the lettuce. Add grated beets, carrots, chopped red cabbage, fennel, celery, and other alkaline raw vegetables. Add alkaline with raw garlic and onions. If you also drink plenty of fresh juices, especially cleansing vegetable juices, substitute "tonics" now and then for a lunch or dinner, and drink herbal

---

we don't use (elimination). Although each of these three functions is always going on to some extent, each is more intense during certain hours of the day:

> noon to 8 P.M.—appropriation (eating and digestion)
> 8 P.M. to 4 A.M.—assimilation (absorption and use)
> 4 A.M. to noon—elimination (of body wastes and food debris)

Our body cycles can become apparent to us if we simply witness our bodies in action. Obviously, during our waking hours we eat (appropriate), and if we put off eating, our hunger tends to heighten as the day goes on. When we are sleeping and the body has no other noticeable work to do, it is assimilating what was taken in during the day. When we awaken in the morning, we have what is called 'morning breath' and perhaps a coated tongue because our bodies are in the midst of eliminating that which was not used—body wastes. . . . Understand that elimination means the removal of toxic waste and excess weight from your body." Harvey and Marilyn Diamond. *Fit for Life*. New York: Warner Books, 1985, pp. 27–28.

teas as often as you can instead of coffee, soda, or caffeinated tea, you may be up to 55 to 60 percent.

Then in the evening, you compatibly combine a greater amount of alkaline vegetables to balance the whole grains, legumes, and proteins you are eating, and you are easily at 75 percent.

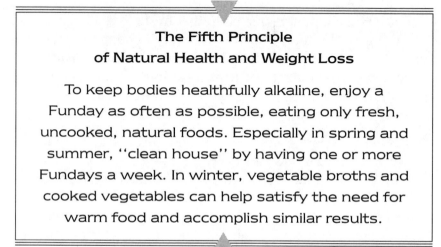

**The Fifth Principle
of Natural Health and Weight Loss**

To keep bodies healthfully alkaline, enjoy a Funday as often as possible, eating only fresh, uncooked, natural foods. Especially in spring and summer, "clean house" by having one or more Fundays a week. In winter, vegetable broths and cooked vegetables can help satisfy the need for warm food and accomplish similar results.

The Alkaline Diet and Weight Loss

We're not trying to drown you in numbers, we're merely showing you how easy it can be to prevent acidosis so that you feel and look your best. This is also, not coincidentally, the same approach that will take off the most weight. The recipes in the FITONICS FORMULA, supported by BODYTONICS and the deep-relaxing breathing in Hypno-Meditation and MIND-TONICS, will help you alkalinize your body.

One of the best ways we have found to lose weight, boost our enzyme counts, and flush acids from our systems is to occasionally have an entire day on live food, a 100 percent alkaline

Funday. To keep ourselves radiant and energetic, we make every effort—especially during the warm months—to have one or more live food days a week. After a day or two like this, we look years younger, feel rested, and are exploding with energy and creativity.

This is particularly easy and agreeable to do as a spring "housecleaning" as warm weather approaches. Alkaline days during the summer *cool* our bodies and flush out heat-generating fats, thus making us more heat-tolerant. An all-juice day, especially in the summer, when we can flush our bodies with luscious and sweet watermelon juice and plenty of vegetable juices, will have the same effect.

In Germany, it has long been a national custom called *gesundheitstag* to eat only one kind of fruit for a full day. Among Natural Health practitioners, that beneficial habit is called "mono-dieting." It allows you to save time and energy by freeing yourself from meal preparation and clean-up. You will be amazed at how many extra hours you gain on the days you chose to eat LIVE FOOD.

Weaning Yourself of Habit-Forming Acids

Acidosis can be blamed for addiction. Tobacco and coffee are acid-forming.

As tobacco and coffee turn your body more and more acidic, you will find yourselves craving them more and more. To break addictions such as these, an alkaline diet certainly can't hurt.[5]

The cigarette habit is a tough one to break. And yet, millions have succeeded in eliminating this deadly habit from their lives. Our friend, Frank, is a stellar example:

---

[5]Rita Romano. *Dining in the Raw: Cooking with the Buff.* Florence, Italy: Nuovo Castello, 1993, p. 25.

Frank is a seventy-one-years-young Irishman from Brooklyn with an unusual passion for people and life. For sixty-three years, up until January 4, 1996, he had been smoking three packs of cigarettes a day.

When we met him in 1995, he had been successful on FIT FOR LIFE and was enthusiastic to learn about FITONICS. He had already lost twenty-five pounds by food combining and eating fruit in the morning. We told him about enzymes and reinforced his fruit and vegetable focus.

Within three weeks of taking alkalinizing plant enzymes and giving up acid-forming sugar and white flour, Frank called one day and told us he was ready to stop smoking. We met again, emphasized the importance of drinking alkaline carrot juice every day, taught Frank BODYTONICS, and shared the MINDTONIC and Hypno-Meditation instructions specific for smoking and weight loss (which you will find in chapters 10 and 11).

Enzymes, live food, juices, deep breathing, changes in thinking and posture, and relaxation all reduced the acidity in Frank's body to allow him to stop smoking. At seventy-one, Frank broke a lifelong habit and became an active champion of Natural Health.

Can I Still Have a Drink?

The question always comes up, and when we look to the Natural Health pioneers for support for alcohol consumption, by and large, *we won't find it!*

Dr. Norman Walker, author of twelve books on Natural Health, who lived *robustly* to age 106, wrote in *Become Younger*[6] that alcohol "acts as a solvent for elements in the body which are only soluble in alcohol and are difficult to rebuild. It tends

---

[6]Norman Walker. *Become Younger*. Prescott, Ariz.: Norwalk Press, 1978, p. 28.

to destroy more or less gradually the texture of the kidneys. It affects the nerves which are closely related to the brain and has the tendency to disrupt the functions of observation, concentration, and locomotion . . ."

Linda Ojeda, Ph.D., author of *Menopause Without Medicine*, tells us that "alcohol hinders the body's ability to absorb several of the B vitamins and disrupts levels of magnesium, potassium and zinc."[7]

We would like to add that since alcohol is so acidic in the body, it disrupts homeostasis, the healthy acid/alkaline balance of your blood. Since alcohol is also a depressant of the central nervous system, it may slow down the movement of food through your digestive tract. The question is, therefore, *how much* to drink, if you enjoy your alcoholic beverage.

We think Dr. Ojeda's further comments answer that question in a most relevant way:

"The French outlive Americans by about 2½ years and suffer 40 percent fewer heart attacks—despite the fact that smoking is a national pastime and their diet swims in a big pool of fat . . .

"Several population studies have suggested that *moderate* amounts of alcohol (one to two drinks per day) may help prevent heart disease. Alcohol appears to help the heart by raising HDLs, decreasing the stickiness of blood platelets, and lowering the levels of fibrinogen, a potent risk factor for heart disease. European researchers have found that red wine contains phenolic compounds, which have strong antioxidant properties that limit the oxidation of LDLs.

"Is it wine that wards off heart attacks in the French, or is it because they eat more fresh fruits and vegetables than Americans, take longer to relish their meals, and use more olive oil and less butter in cooking? In other words, is it because their *entire* lifestyle is more stress-free than that of the typical Ameri-

---

[7]Linda Ojeda. *Menopause Without Medicine*. Alameda, Calif.: Hunter House, 1992, p. 182.

can? When headlines sensationalize one food or substance and label it a 'cure,' it is important to realize that, when it comes to disease and health, many factors participate."

We cannot agree with Dr. Ojeda more when she stresses *moderation* in alcohol intake. We would also add that the French have such a high ethic about quality food, they consume far less junk, processed food, and sugar than Americans.

The effects of alcohol in the body cannot be minimized. More than three glasses a day can:

▶ Raise your blood pressure

▶ Reduce the flow of blood to your heart

▶ Cause irregular heartbeats

▶ Raise blood triglyceride levels

▶ Ultimately damage the heart muscle

▶ Unhealthfully acidify your bloodstream

▶ Contribute to sleeplessness, weight gain, and nervous tension from poor digestion, and a slowing of the elimination process

▶ Increase the risk of breast cancer

▶ Damage the liver

All of this information correlates with Natural Health guidelines to keep your alcohol intake to a minimum as you *increase* your intake of water and fresh juices. If your goal is weight loss, remember that alcohol provides *no* nutrition. Only empty calories! And remember that increased triglycerides mean more fat stored on your waist, hips and thighs.

So how do you have a rich social experience if alcohol is, for you—as it is for most people—part of the art of relaxation, gourmet eating, football fun, and celebrations?

► Cut "down" rather than "out." For wellness, depending on your size, and whether you are a man or a woman, limit your alcohol intake to ONE SHOT a day. There's a folklore in Europe and China that a shot a day of pure, *high-quality* spirits is actually good for your health. This would include a good whiskey or a fine wine or beer.

► If you enjoy red wine, use the French custom for giving wine to young children at celebrations, *dilute it.* Order a glass of red wine and pour a little of it in your ice water.

► Add a half shot rather than a whole shot of bourbon to your soda.

► Reserve your alcohol intake for weekends.

► Avoid the mixed drinks with syrups and sugar that carry fancy names and high price tags.

► Opt for drinking pure water *enzymized* with lemon or lime.

Many people have parents or grandparents who have embraced the tradition of a shot a day and lived to ripe old ages healthfully. Excess, of course, cannot be life-extending, for all the reasons we have mentioned. And, *of course*, if you have heart, liver, or kidney problems and your doctor has recommended abstention, you'd be foolish not to listen!

And keep in mind that alcohol is *dehydrating*. In all likelihood you've experienced this truth when you've awakened after a "bash" to a dry mouth and throat. So, when you do drink alcohol, be sure to increase your water intake.

If you, too, want to become a champion of Natural Health, it is important for you to know that one of the most treacherous acid-forming foods in your diet is . . .

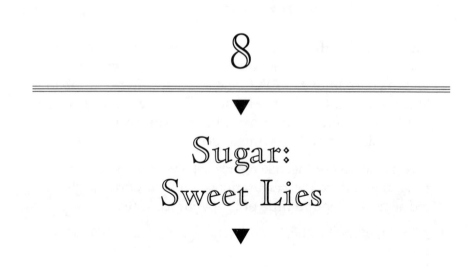

8

Sugar:
Sweet Lies

▼

Human beings have a naturally sweet palate. Mother's milk is sweet. Throughout the ages, our natural sweet has been fruit. Two hundred years ago, much to our detriment, that story changed. That's when the process of sugar refinement began to transform our diets.

We have a sense you know what we're about to say: *IT'S THE REFINED SUGAR YOU EAT THAT MAKES YOU FAT.* You *know* this! Perhaps you don't know, however, that it's that same sugar when you eat it with fat, carbohydrates, or protein, that makes you even fatter.

We are talking about all refined sugar from the sugarcane and sugar beet industries. This includes refined white sugar, powdered sugar, brown sugar, and turbinado sugar. The fact is, Americans consume nearly 125 pounds of sugar for every man, woman, and child per year.[1]

You may have been told that it is calories that make you fat

[1]Gabriel Cousens. *Conscious Eating*. Santa Rosa, Calif.: Vision Books International, 1992, p. 91.

and that you can have sugar as long as your total caloric intake is low enough. The low-fat and fat-free industries that replace the naturally occurring fats in foods such as dairy with *unnatural* sugar thrive on this bit of mythology. If you believe it, you may also be willing to consider that hemlock is good for you, too, as long as you keep your calories budgeted.

Sugar is hidden in practically everything you buy in the supermarket. It is what is known as a *cheap filler.* That's fairly self-explanatory. It's the old game of giving *nothing* and charging for it.

The Hidden Killer

William Dufty's prophetic book, *Sugar Blues,* warned us about the powerful economic interests of the sugar industry: "The sugar industry has invested millions of dollars in behind-the-scenes, subsidized science to convince the public that sugar is a harmless 'fun-food.' "[2]

"It has been proven, however, that (1) sugar is a major factor in dental decay; (2) sugar in a person's diet does cause overweight; (3) removal of sugar from diets has cured symptoms of crippling, and diseases such as diabetes, cancer and heart illness."[3]

Traditional medical science seems to actually suppress the truth about sugar. One obvious example is the focus on fluoride to "fight" tooth decay. What a smoke screen! We add a profitable and potentially carcinogenic[4] by-product from industry in our water in order to "prevent" cavities rather than removing sugar from our diets and from all the processed foods to which it is routinely added.

---

[2]A frequently quoted party line coming from such prestigious schools of nutrition as Harvard.

[3]William Dufty. *Sugar Blues.* New York: Warner Books, 1975, pp. 138–39.

[4]"The Fluoride Risk: Evidence of a Link to Cancer." *Newsweek,* February 5, 1990.

Dufty's report of further suppressive shenanigans is anything but sweet: "During the nineteenth century, the incidence of diabetes seemed to increase over that of ancient times. Figures relating to the consumption of sugar in early America to the number of deaths from diabetes have not been compiled. Denmark has such statistics, but medical histories in the U.S. rarely mention them, or make any connection between sugar and diabetes . . ."[5] Dufty's conclusion is inescapable: "As sugar consumption escalates wildly, fatal diseases increase remorselessly."[6]

It is interesting that the level of diabetes has increased 50 percent since 1983 and has tripled since 1958. Eleven million people suffered from the disease in 1983; 16 million are afflicted today. This disheartening statistic applies to Type II diabetes, the form that makes up 95 percent of all cases and can be prevented and controlled with diet.[7] This form is related to obesity, and it leads to potential blindness and early death.

> "In one small study at Loma Linda University, researchers gave participants 100 grams of sugar (three cans of soda) and then watched as their neutrophil (immune activity) sank about 45 percent. Five hours later it was still substantially below normal."
>
> —*Fitness*, January-February 1996

We relate this increase in incidence to increased sugar consumption and to the advent of the low-fat industry, which removes fat from food and replaces it, in a large number of cases, with sugar. Sugar is added to a plethora of commonly consumed junk foods that were not even available in the 1950s, and we find it in all sorts of foods that don't require it. In the last five years, Americans have consumed more candy than ever before in history—an average of twenty-one pounds a person annually.[8]

In some of their books, Natural Health pioneers Drs. Paul

---

[5]Dufty. *Sugar Blues*, p. 79.
[6]Ibid., p. 79.
[7]Dr. Richard Eastman. National Institute of Diabetes and Digestive and Kidney Diseases, reported in *Arizona Republic*, November 3, 1995, p. A6.
[8]*Parade*, November 12, 1995, p. 5.

and Virginia Bragg wrote about Dr. Robert McCracken, a UCLA anthropologist. Dr. McCracken concluded from his research that humans are naturally fruit, vegetable, and meat eaters. Our grain consumption began only approximately 10,000 years ago. Our refined sugar habit is merely a few centuries old. He believed that ancient man was healthier than modern man.

Dr. McCracken faulted refined sugar to a large extent for some forms of diabetes, heart disease, stroke, schizophrenia, alcoholism, and even possibly some kinds of cancer.[9] McCracken noted that members of certain primitive tribes who consume many more saturated fats than Americans, who never touch refined sugar, have normal blood cholesterol levels and few of the diseases to which we fall victim.

What Really Happens When You Eat Sugar?

We Americans have finally come to the point in nutritional evolution where we want the truth. The knowledge you are seeking is the power that will allow you to make a change. Here's the scoop on what happens when you eat sugar:

The biggest problem your body faces each time refined sugar is taken into it is the rapid rate of absorption. Sugar rushes through the stomach wall without being digested, stimulating excess secretion of the powerful hormone insulin by the pancreas and causing metabolic imbalances.

As the sugar enters your bloodstream, insulin is immediately secreted by the pancreas to facilitate its passage through the cell membrane to your tissues, where it is used as fuel. That sounds innocent enough, but in a moment you'll understand why you would *never* want that to happen.

---

[9]Paul Bragg and Virginia Bragg. *Healthy Eating Without Confusion.* Santa Barbara, Calif.: Health Science, 1967, p. 12.

As you have learned, your pancreas is the organ largely responsible for manufacturing your enzymes. In a previous chapter, we pointed out that in most Americans the pancreas is so overworked it is enlarged far beyond its normal size. One of the reasons the pancreas may be enlarged, aside from the continuous demand being made on it for enzyme production (one and a half liters a day of digestive juices), is the massive dose of sugar it is frequently being forced to deal with each day.

The daily average for sugar consumption is a third of a pound for every man, woman, and child. That amounts to approximately five ounces, or over half a cup of sugar every day. And there are many who are eating so much more than five ounces a day.

Could you sit down with a spoon and eat more than half a cup of sugar? Mouthful after mouthful? We don't think so. However, this is, in fact, what millions of men, women, and children are doing, day in and day out—only they're taking it concealed in other foods.

Sabotaging the Brain

Insulin secreted to deal with refined sugar ironically causes your blood sugar level *to fall*. This dramatically affects your brain since it is a very sensitive biochemical organ, operating in a very fine biochemical balance, in which fully 25 percent of the adult body's metabolic activity takes place. When your blood sugar gets too low, as it does when large amounts of insulin are secreted to control the rapidly absorbed refined white sugar, your brain begins to malfunction. It freaks out![10]

Think for a minute of some of the little children you've seen in supermarkets, airports, or shopping malls, wailing pathetically, noses running, tears streaming down their faces, their

---

[10]Ibid., p. 14.

parents harassed and unknowing that it might have been the sugar in their breakfast cereal and the Coke or Pepsi they drank earlier that has them emotionally out of control.

Not only does sugar's effect on the brain seem to be creating problems for small children and their parents, it also has been proved to have significant impact on teenage behavior.

Consistent research findings on teenage offenders show that when their diets were changed from the typical high white sugar and fast food diet, there was a marked *decrease* in the teens' acting out of violent behavior. . . . A two-year, scientifically precise study with 267 subjects by Steven Schoenthaler, Ph.D., published in the *Journal of Biosocial Research*, showed that while the average American eats approximately 125 pounds of sugar, *teenage delinquents consume* **300 pounds per year.** When this sugar intake was significantly reduced . . . and fruits and vegetables were increased, there was a 48 percent decrease in antisocial behavior of all types, including violent crimes, crimes against property, and runaways. This was true for all ages and races.[11]

EMILY

Emily is an adorable, highly intelligent, blond seven-year-old who took part in one of our FITONICS groups in 1994. She was a choosy eater, and her loving parents were always trying to entice her to pick up her fork and put "something" into her mouth—until dessert was put in front of her. Then we noticed that Emily immediately showed an interest in eating. But afterward, there were mood swings and sometimes disruptive outbursts that were particularly uncharacteristic.

One day we suggested to Emily that she give up sugar for a while. "Why?" she asked softly, her eyes wide with curiosity.

"Because we think you'll be happier without it, Emmy."

---

[11]Ibid., p. 14.

*Our suggestion was enough for Emily. She is an exception-
ally intelligent little child, and she trusted what we told her.*

*"Okay," she said, "I'll try it. But does that mean I can never
have sugar again?"*

*"No," we assured her. "Have it once a month or at special
events like parties."*

*Her parents told us Emily announced the very next day
that she was giving up sugar. She began commenting about
how "unhappy" some of her classmates were after sugary
snacks at school. Even when she attended parties, her parents
reported that she still didn't succumb. She became so commit-
ted, she asked her mother to tell her if sugar was hidden in
something she was eating, and when she found out there was
sugar in the buns at McDonald's, she stopped eating Big Macs.*

*Then came Halloween. Emily hadn't had sugar in six
weeks. After trick-or-treating, she decided this was the "special, once a month" occasion. She ate four pieces of her candy,
and within an hour, she felt miserable.*

*"I'll never eat sugar again," she told her daddy. "I hate the
way it makes me feel."*

Emily may be someone whose individual body chemistry
made her particularly sensitive to sugar. But we believe that
anyone can benefit from controlling sugar intake. The emotional balance, good health, and weight loss that can result are astoundingly dra-
matic.

The brain is the control
system for your entire body.
It gets shortchanged on fuel
when you eat sugar. In this
state of deprivation, it becomes confused, irritated,
restless, and tired. Does that
sound to you like some of

"Researchers at Harvard Medical School
discovered that in order to fatten mice
rapidly, they had to induce brain lesions
by administering continuous doses of
sugar. There is strong evidence recorded
in the periodical literature that heavy use
of refined sugar causes pituitary lesions
and brain lesions like those produced in
the study of mice."

—Edward Howell, *Enzyme Nutrition*

the behavior grade school teachers are reporting? Does it sound like the unexpected emotional outburst or irritability that someone you love demonstrates?

Perhaps you may be wondering how we can say that sugar consumption makes you tired, since its first effect is that rush of energy as it spills into your bloodstream. The answer is simple. Sugar increases the level of serotonin in the brain. Serotonin is the chemical that makes you ready for sleep. That is why you may find yourself craving something sweet when you are upset. You are trying to calm yourself down and knock yourself unconscious in order not to feel your burdens.

Running on Empty

The moment the insulin reaction has cleaned your bloodstream of sugar, your body is suddenly running on empty because sugar does not carry any nutrients. The cells have burned it as fuel, but they've not been nourished. All the vitamins and minerals, the complex carbohydrates, have been stripped away during the refining process. Therefore, when the sugar is out of your system, hunger is felt, along with cravings, and since you are dealing with an addictive substance, those cravings will usually be for something with more sugar . . . like a cookie or a candy bar. And once you satisfy this craving, the vicious cycle of fat storing starts all over again.

Removing Refined Sugar from Your Diet Will Help You Lose Weight and Keep It Off

Here's why. Once your pancreas receives the red alert for too much sugar, and releases insulin, three events happen:

▶ Insulin gives the sugar to your cells to incinerate.

▶ Whatever can't be burned is turned into glycogen, which is a fancy word for stored sugar in the muscles and liver.

▶ The pancreas converts the remaining sugar into triglycerides, another fancy name that might as well mean, "Soon to be worn as body fat on your thighs and belly."

At the start of this chapter, we stated that sugar eaten with fat, carbohydrates, or protein makes you fat. When carbohydrates, fats, and proteins are metabolized they become sugars, free fatty acids, and amino acids circulating in your bloodstream.

Remember, sugar is rapidly absorbed and processed: this means that once sugar has saturated your bloodstream, giving temporary energy, your body has to do something with all the protein, fats, and carbohydrates you consumed. It has no other option but to convert these nutrients to body fat. Please keep this in mind:

ONCE YOU EAT SUGAR,
ALL FAT BURNING COMES TO A STOP!

Why? The abrupt insulin reaction is your body's effort to save itself from sugar poisoning. Excess sugar in the bloodstream is very dangerous, as any diabetic knows. It can lead to cellular dehydration and put you into a potentially fatal coma. Insulin to the rescue! It does its job of making sure the sugar is burned. But you don't want to burn sugar if your goal is to burn fat off your body!

We believe we've made a strong enough case to at least convince you that sugar is definitely not your friend. Here's the icing on the cake:

Refined Sugar Contributes to Constipation

The energy sugar takes from your body has to come from somewhere. We've already discussed in a previous chapter that when your body has to borrow energy, it does so from elimination. In addition, refined sugar lacks fiber—and without fiber, food can't move freely through your digestive tract. Since you will usually find refined sugar combined with other ingredients that lack fiber, such as refined white flour, you are in "double trouble."

Take this test if you need proof. As much as possible avoid all refined sugar in the foods you eat for three days. You can replace your craving for sweets with natural fruit sweetness by having the following:

▶ An ample fruit breakfast that includes some dates or dried fruit. (See fruit cereal recipes.)

▶ A fruit snack during the mid-morning hours.

▶ A large sweet carrot or fresh fruit juice before lunch. (This very alkaline juice will help neutralize the acid in your body that is leading you to crave acid foods like sugar.)

▶ Small amounts of sun-dried fruits, such as bananas, figs, raisins, or dates. (Sulfur-dried fruits are acidic and can cause stomach upset.)

▶ Half a cantaloupe or honeydew or a grapefruit before dinner.

▶ A banana before bed.

After your three-day "fast" from refined sugar, you may notice a predictable benefit from eating so much fruit sugar. Your elimination process will undoubtedly have improved. In addition, you might notice you're actually feeling quite energized and even-tempered.

Now, take the experiment one step further. For supper, eat a good-sized sugary dessert. What happens in the morning! NOT MUCH! Elimination, we mean. And, perhaps, a feeling of irritability because you have not fully rested. And you may wake up hungry. The sugar has robbed your body of essential (alkaline) nutrients it wants you to quickly replace.

> **Sugar can weaken the immune system**
>
> "Dr. Joseph Pizzorno, N.D., president of Bastyr University of Naturopathic Medicine, says as little as 100 grams at one sitting (the equivalent of a 5-ounce chocolate bar and a can of soda) can suppress your immune system for up to six hours."
>
> —*Self*, January 1996

If you have a sweet tooth, join the rest of us. That sweet tooth is perfectly natural. Don't feel you have to apologize for it! You inherited it! Your primitive ancestors, the hunter-gatherers, essentially lived on sweet plant food and fatty animal food. They had to in order to survive and ensure nutrient and energy reserves in times of scarcity. But . . . their primary sources of sweet foods were fruits and roots. There were no "Snickers trees."

Healthy Substitutes for Refined Sugar

Your natural craving for sweet foods has been artificially perverted by the eating of refined sugar. But you can turn that around. What is more important to you—your normal slender weight and good health, or a candy bar?

Nature provided plenty of natural sugar sources by giving us a cornucopia of fruits. They will take weight off, not put it on!

In addition, the natural food industry now produces many healthful and natural whole-food sweeteners such as raw honey,[12] concentrated fruit juice, pure maple syrup, brown rice syrup, sorghum, and date sugar.

There are many unrefined sweeteners like date sugar, rice sugar, and dehydrated cane juice which can be easily substituted, measure for measure, in any recipe calling for white sugar. Sometimes, the finished product will have a slightly golden, more natural color, but consistency and moisture will not change.

Many health-conscious mothers are now choosing natural sweeteners made from fresh-cut, organically grown sugarcane. One such product is Sucanat®. When it is produced, the juice is pressed from the cane, concentrated, and then dehydrated into a crystalline powder resembling dry brown sugar. It retains nutritious minerals (calcium, iron, magnesium, phosphorus, and potassium), vitamins (A, C, B_1, B_2, and B_6), and trace elements (chromium, copper, and zinc). All these nutrients are found in natural sugarcane, and all are removed during the refining of white, brown, and turbinado sugar.

> "To rev up your immune system, reduce your sweets and pile on the fruits and vegetables."
> —*Fitness*, January-February 1996

Our favorite sweeteners in baking are date sugar for the fiber it supplies and Sucanat.

Anyone Out There Still Not Convinced?

Dr. Nancy Appleton, author of *Lick the Sugar Habit*, gives us fifty-nine reasons why sugar ruins our health, each one backed up by references from medical journals, books, and periodicals.

---

[12]Raw honey is more healthful than honey that is heated because it contains enzymes.

59 REASONS WHY SUGAR
RUINS OUR HEALTH

1. Can suppress the immune system.
2. Can upset the minerals in the body.
3. Can cause hyperactivity, anxiety, difficulty concentrating, and crankiness in children.
4. Produces a significant rise in triglycerides.
5. Contributes to the reduction in defense against bacterial infection.
6. Can cause kidney damage.
7. Reduces high-density lipoproteins.
8. Leads to chromium deficiency.
9. Leads to cancer of the breast, ovaries, intestines, prostate, and rectum.
10. Increases fasting levels of glucose and insulin.
11. Causes a copper deficiency.
12. Interferes with absorption of calcium and magnesium.
13. Weakens eyesight.
14. Raises the level of neurotransmitters called serotonin.
15. Can cause hypoglycemia.
16. Can produce an acidic stomach.
17. Can raise adrenaline levels in children.
18. Malabsorption is frequent in patients with functional bowel disease.
19. Can cause aging.
20. Can lead to alcoholism.
21. Can cause tooth decay.
22. Contributes to obesity.
23. Increases the risk of Crohn's disease and ulcerative colitis.
24. Can cause changes frequently found in people with gastric or duodenal ulcers.
25. Can cause arthritis.
26. Can cause asthma.
27. Can cause *Candida albicans* (yeast infections).
28. Can cause gallstones.

29. Can cause heart disease.
30. Can cause appendicitis.
31. Can cause multiple sclerosis.
32. Can cause hemorrhoids.
33. Can cause varicose veins.
34. Can elevate glucose and insulin responses in oral contraceptive users.
35. Can lead to periodontal disease.
36. Can contribute to osteoporosis.
37. Contributes to saliva acidity.
38. Can cause a decrease in insulin sensitivity.
39. Leads to decreased glucose intolerance.
40. Can decrease growth hormone.
41. Can increase cholesterol.
42. Can increase the systolic blood pressure.
43. Can cause drowsiness and decreased activity in children.
44. Can cause migraine headaches.
45. Can interfere with the absorption of protein.
46. Causes food allergies.
47. Can contribute to diabetes.
48. Can cause toxemia during pregnancy.
49. Can contribute to eczema in children.
50. Can cause cardiovascular disease.
51. Can impair the structure of DNA.
52. Can change the structure of protein.
53. Can make your skin age by changing the structure of collagen.
54. Can cause cataracts.
55. Can cause emphysema.
56. Can cause atherosclerosis.
57. Can promote an elevation of low-density lipoprotein (LDL).
58. Can cause free radicals in the bloodstream.
59. *LOWERS THE ENZYMES' ABILITY TO FUNCTION.*[13]

---

[13]*Health Freedom News*, June 1994.

We're on Your Side!

FITONICS has been designed to help you move away from a sugar habit. Of course, you will, on occasion, eat a little sugar. After all, your loved ones will have birthdays. And sometimes it will unavoidably be a minor ingredient in some supermarket foods.

But overall, from day to day, you can break the "habit." Take advantage of all the delicious, sweet juice blends and tonics, your morning fruit "cereals," dried fruits, fruit platters for lunch, or an evening fruit meal that will go a long way toward satisfying your sugar craving. They'll answer the deeper biological need for sweets, formed at the origin of our history as a species, with the foods we used then to satisfy it.

But . . . be on your guard. Don't believe "sugar-coated" advertising. The mainstream food industry is not on your side. Remember, sugar is one of its cheapest fillers, and since it is also addicting, it is used in everything. Even ketchup! Children are particularly targeted on morning television with products that frequently contain up to three teaspoons or more of sugar per serving. The new trend to "frost" all cereals, even Cheerios, is just one more chilling example of the profit, rather than health, motivations in the cereal industry.[14]

The number of overweight children in our country has doubled since the 1960s. As of November 1995, 6.7 million children ages six to seventeen are overweight. A nation's wealth is its children. A shocking 11 percent of those we want to nurture and cherish are now saddled with the disability of excess weight. Is it any wonder when 91 percent of foods advertised on television to children are high in fat, sugar, and salt?[15]

---

[14]Such foods as cereal, ketchup, salad dressing, mayonnaise, and soft drinks, which routinely have added sugar, can be found sugar-free or with healthy sweeteners in natural food stores.

[15]*Tufts University Diet and Nutrition Letter*, November 1995, p. 2.

Bravo! Nabisco!

Finally, a cereal manufacturer is providing us with a truly good-tasting, high-fiber, sugar-free cereal: Mini-Shredded Wheat with Bran. Toss in some raisins and banana, pour on the soy milk, and enjoy a wonderful, healthful meal, morning, noon, or night.

While thousands of medical research papers make the strongest case possible for eating fiber to lower our obesity statistics, cure our constipation, and thereby decrease the risk of cancer and heart disease, most cereal makers still cater exclusively to the sweet palate, continuing to add fattening sugar rather than slenderizing, fiber-rich whole grains to their products.

Cereal is one of the most important sources for fiber, and a huge number of us are ready for more American food manufacturers to step up to the plate and produce for us truly high-fiber cereals that taste good without sugar. Even those cereals advertised as "high-fiber" yield only a pitiful one or two grams of fiber per serving. A bona fide high-fiber cereal should have five to ten grams of fiber per serving!

> "The trick of losing weight is to get the most satisfaction from the fewest calories. The most satiating foods are those high in fiber, especially such fruits as apples and oranges. Potatoes top the list for fullness, as do whole grains. Fish outperforms steak. Foods high in fat are the least filling (you have to eat much more of them)—and those highest in fat and sugar are the least satiating because only a small portion of nutrients [enter the body] with a high number of calories."
> —*Environmental Nutrition*, February 1996

Until you move away from sugar, you will never realize how much pain and suffering it is causing your body and your mind. Try pure, whole alternative sweeteners. For a wonderful life of health and happiness, eat real, nutritious foods and avoid such phonies as . . .

9

Aspartame and Olestra: The Shuck and the Jive

First, the "shuck." This is the story of something that looks like sugar, supposedly tastes like sugar (although it's 180 to 200 times sweeter), and even feels like sugar. Developed by the B. D. Searle pharmaceutical company, it was initially marketed to the public as a safe, calorie-free sugar substitute in advertisements touting it as "natural" as a glass of milk and a banana, as if it comes from something so natural as a piece of fruit or an animal.

Years later, that ad campaign is still working. Under the brand names of NutraSweet and Equal, aspartame is consumed several times a day by over 100 million Americans who think they are doing something good for themselves.

Aspartame and Soft Drinks

The food-manufacturing and pharmaceutical industries love aspartame. It's found in everything from cola to coffee cake, cereals to children's vitamin supplements. There's hardly a packaged food that doesn't contain it, and nowhere is it more prevalent than in the soft drink industry. We're guzzling so much aspartame in this country, one would think it flowed directly from heaven, via the clouds that bring us our rain, into our snow-fed streams, lakes, and rivers.

Only the terrible distance between us and our natural instincts to survive can explain how an entire population, one third of which is overweight and growing more so, could swallow the scientifically promoted idea that we can take a pharmaceutical chemical into our bodies to fool our sweet-craving taste buds and not do any damage. But we're buying it!

When aspartame was introduced under the brand Nutra-Sweet, diet drink consumption went up six times. In 1985, we were ingesting 800 million pounds of aspartame-sweetened soft drinks, a figure that has assuredly doubled by now.

How could that have been possible? It's no accident. There is an addictive quality to aspartame, just as there is to sugar. *And* . . . ASPARTAME CREATES INCREASED THIRST. That may now explain to you why having just one of these drinks is never enough. You have one, and you may find yourself drinking them all day long.

Debunking the Dangerous Mythology of Aspartame

Now here's the "bitter" truth. Aspartame is not a product derived from bananas or cows. It's a totally synthetic chemical additive *manufactured in a laboratory*. There are numerous studies, in all probability funded by the manufacturers, reporting "no conclusive evidence" that aspartame is harmful. How can it be explained, then, that this one chemical has prompted the longest list of complaints ever received by the FDA?

The very nature of aspartame and what it does in the body is the answer to that question. The chemical is composed of three ingredients that occur naturally but are never found in combination in nature. When you eat aspartame, you are eating two amino acids (phenylalanine and aspartic acid) and methanol (methyl alcohol). (Does your common sense tell you right away that that is not how nature intended for you to satisfy your natural craving for sweet?)

After entering the body, the three components of aspartame are rapidly released into your bloodstream. Methanol, a deadly poison that is rarely found in free form, is the first to be separated. It can cause serious tissue damage. Some of the symptoms of methanol poisoning are headaches; numbness of the arms, hands, legs, or feet; dizziness; depression; blurred vision; nausea; and stomach pain. At high levels, methanol attacks the retina of the eye, causing blindness.

Pregnant women, in particular, are warned by many doctors to avoid aspartame because high methanol levels can result in lack of formation of the eyes of their child. High levels of intake during pregnancy have been associated with a 10 to 15 percent drop in IQ levels in infants. Yet how many products containing the chemical offer this warning?

One of the reasons methanol is so toxic is because your body lacks the specific *enzymes* necessary to detoxify it. The amount of time it requires to be eliminated from your body is five times the elimination time required for the ethyl alcohol in beer, whiskey, or wine. If aspartame is heated above 85 degrees, which can happen routinely during warehousing and delivery, or even if you keep cases of aspartame-sweetened beverages in your garage, the product itself decomposes, resulting in freestanding methanol.[1]

Which means that when you open a can of diet soda to quench your thirst, you're drinking a virulent poison. Before aspartame is eliminated, your body must go through an energy-draining conversion process, one stage of which results in the conversion of the methanol to formaldehyde. Formaldehyde is used for embalming!

---

[1]David Steinman. *Diet for a Poisoned Planet*. New York: Ballantine Books, 1990, p. 190.

We need to take the hint! Why would you ever want to put anything into your body that causes formaldehyde formation? One twelve-ounce can of aspartame-sweetened diet beverage contains about ten milligrams of NutraSweet. Heavy consumers of diet beverages could be easily taking in one hundred milligrams a day, which is thirteen times the limit recommended as safe by the Environmental Protection Agency.

The Threat May Be Even More Serious Than We Thought

Although the relative concentration of phenylalanine and aspartic acid is ten times higher than that found naturally in foods, literature distributed by the industry to promote aspartame products suggests that the body treats these two amino acids as if they were coming from fruit, vegetable, milk, or meat sources. That's like saying that smog has the same sweet effect in our lungs as the air in a giant redwood forest!

Dr. H. J. Roberts, a physician and aspartame researcher, explains that when these amino acids are consumed in their natural state in foods, they are digested and released into your bloodstream slowly, buffered and balanced by other amino acids. However, especially when aspartame is consumed in beverages, your body is suddenly flooded with phenylalanine and aspartic acid, which can cross into the brain unimpeded and cause "significant disturbances."

Dr. Roberts is an exceptional physician. He has published more than two hundred articles and letters in leading medical journals and has written five books, including the highly respected medical text *Difficult Diagnosis: A Guide to the Interpretation of Severe Illness*. In his recent book, *Aspartame (NutraSweet): Is It Safe?*, he states, "Aspartame is potentially dangerous and may produce a wide variety of physical and mental symptoms, most of which now go unrecognized or are misinterpreted as serious illness."

Soon after the introduction of aspartame to the marketplace, Roberts noticed clusters of symptoms that were difficult to diagnose and treat. These included: headaches, dizziness and unsteadiness, confusion and memory loss, decreased vision, severe depression, extreme irritability, severe anxiety attacks, severe drowsiness, marked personality change, palpitations, tachycardia, tingling, convulsions, nausea, severe insomnia, ringing in the ears, diarrhea, frequency of urination accompanied by burning, excessive thirst, severe slurring of speech, and severe joint pains.

Here's where we arrive at the crux of our problem. The symptoms Dr. Roberts relates to the introduction of aspartame are most frequently brought to the attention of a physician, who may unknowingly misdiagnose them as one form of disease or another. The symptoms are then treated with other drugs, which often add additional side effects, at great expense to you, the patient.

This is a flagrant example of a terrible injustice: So much of what is added to your food, beyond your control, is contributing to much of the serious illness that is crippling our society. Many doctors and Natural Health advocates spoke out against aspartame when it was approved by the commissioner of the FDA in 1981. Yet the commissioner was known to have *deliberately* overruled the warnings from a federally appointed board of inquiry that approval be denied. These official warnings were made after significant indications that aspartame caused brain tumors.

Those Who Spoke Out

Dissenting FDA scientist Dr. Robert Condon wrote in an internal government document in 1981: "I do not concur that aspartame has been shown safe with respect to the induction of brain tumors."[2] Other scientists, among them Dr. Richard Wurtman, professor of neuroendocrinology at MIT, raised serious questions about the sweetener's safety.

As a result, the FDA created a public board of inquiry to examine the results of one hundred tests Searle had submitted to the agency in the 1970s. The board, headed by Walle Nauta, a professor of psychology and brain science at MIT, recommended against the approval of NutraSweet. This is the decision the FDA commissioner overturned.

How did this happen? What lobby prevailed? Certainly none representing *your* well-being and the health of those you love.

The Greatest Irony of All

If you are using aspartame products to lose weight, you should know that's like punching a hole in the bottom of your dinghy. Normally, a meal including carbohydrates will result in a satiated feeling. This is, in part, due to the serotonin production we discussed in the last chapter.

Aspartame is a phony! It only masquerades as a carbohydrate. It has the opposite effect. If you add it to a meal—in a diet soda, coffee, or tea—or if it is the sweetener used by industry in one of the foods you have eaten, all serotonin production in the brain comes to a stop. You don't feel satisfied at all. You want more food, and so you keep eating.

And since you might have bought industry's claims that low-calorie foods take the weight off, you reach for more food sweetened with aspartame. You're in a vicious cycle, flooding

---

[2]Ibid., p. 192.

your body with poisonous methanol, signing up for all the potential symptoms and side effects, and struggling with a weight problem no amount of low-calorie food seems to lick.

The Sixth Principle
of Natural Health and Weight Loss

Think twice before using
sugar and artificial ingredients.

Get Real!

Now, the jive. While we're on the subject of phonies, let's take a moment to put olestra where it belongs . . . which is *anywhere* but in your body.

Major consumer and health groups, including the American Public Health Association, the University of California School of Public Health, the National Women's Health Network, the American Academy of Ophthalmology, and the Center for Science in the Public Interest, have come out against approval of olestra. Despite extensive clinical trials on humans and animals and hundreds of thousands of pages of studies, experts argue that there are no assurances that this controversial, indigestible fat substitute won't ultimately pose a significant danger to your health.

Dr. Sheldon Margen, professor emeritus of public health nutrition at UC Berkeley and chairman of the editorial board of the *UC Berkeley Wellness Letter*, tells us that "the physical properties of olestra are virtually identical to mineral oil and petrolatum."[3] Mineral oil, Dr. Margen explains, is a laxative that carries

---

[3]*UC Berkeley Wellness Letter*, February 1996, p. 2.

a warning against long-term usage "because of its effects on nutrients, the risk of laxative dependence, and other potential adverse effects."[4]

In scientific research on fat-free cookies made with mineral oil, symptoms of gas, bloating, diarrhea, and rectal leakage have continuously been reported. Dr. Margen's conclusion: "The evidence for potentially adverse effects from olestra is overwhelming."[5] Rectal leakage? Anyone telling us that some new miracle food causes rectal leakage is "jivin'" us about the food aspect.

"I don't think this substance should be in the food supply," says Joan Gussow, a Columbia University nutritionist. "Would we put something in the water supply that caused this harm?"[6]

Echoing this sentiment is Michael Jacobson, the executive director of the Center for Science in the Public Interest: " 'It's crazy to add a substance to the food supply that makes people sick.' Jacobson predicts that if olestra is allowed on the market, it will bring an epidemic of diarrhea, cramps and gastrointestinal effects."[7]

Dr. Meir Stampfer, a professor of epidemiology at Harvard University, is among the many scientists who lament olestra's depletion of nutrients from the body—nutrients that reduce the risk of cancer. He says that allowing olestra into the American diet would be "appalling." We couldn't agree more.

Dr. Henry Blackburn, a professor of public health at the University of Minnesota, said olestra failed to meet the FDA's standard of "reasonable certainty of no harm."[8] Then how did it win approval?

Can a fake fat actually help you lose weight? Let's look at what we already know. Fake sugar hasn't made a dent in our

---

[4]Ibid.
[5]Ibid.
[6]Steve Wilson. *Arizona Republic*, "Fat Substitute a Milestone, but May Chip Away Nutrition." November 19, 1995.
[7]Ibid.
[8]Ibid.

weight tables. Since 1981, and the approval of NutraSweet, our obesity statistics have only increased. Dr. Michael Hamilton, the director of the Duke University Diet and Fitness Center, says, "NutraSweet was heralded as the great savior for the overweight, but studies have shown that people who eat foods with NutraSweet eat something else to compensate for the lost calories."

When olestra does make it into your chips and cookies, you should keep one subtle factor in mind: Although those snacks will be fat-free, they won't be calorie-free. It's fairly common knowledge now that when people are eating fat-free they have a tendency to eat more. So your fat-free snack could easily end up being high-calorie.

Again, notwithstanding so much scientific uproar and a considerable amount of commonsense argument, the FDA has given approval to a product that "no one can be certain won't be a danger to public health."[9] Why? Is it perhaps because of the $200,000,000 spent by Procter & Gamble to develop olestra? It might interest you to know that the FDA has no money to fund its own research on such a controversial product. It is forced to rely on the *only* studies done—those funded by Procter & Gamble.

One of the longest such studies, lasting thirty-nine weeks, used pigs for subjects. Dr. Walter Willett, the chairman of the Department of Nutrition at Harvard University School of Public Health, has a classic comment: "They want to give something to my kids on the basis of studying pigs."[10]

If all of this makes you feel like Alice Through the Looking Glass, we believe you're ready for . . .

---

[9]Michael D. Lemonick. *Time*, "Are We Ready for Fat-Free Fat?" January 8, 1996.
[10]Ibid.

PART TWO

BREAKTHROUGH THINKING

10

▼

MINDTONICS:
Optimistic Thinking . . .
and So Much More

▼

Optimism

Talk happiness. The world is sad enough
Without your woes. No path is wholly rough;
Look for the places that are smooth and clear,
And speak of those, to rest the weary ear
Of Earth, so hurt by one continuous strain
Of human discontent and grief and pain.

Talk Faith. The world is better off without
Your uttered ignorance and morbid doubt.
If you have faith in God, or man, or self,
Say so. If not, push back upon the shelf
Of silence all your thoughts, till faith shall come;
No one will grieve because your lips are dumb.

Talk health. The dreary never-changing tale
Of mortal maladies is worn and stale.
You cannot charm, or interest, or please
By harping on that minor chord disease.
Say you are well, or all is well with you.
And God shall hear your words and make them true.
                                          —ELLA WHEELER WILCOX

Are you aware of the tremendous role your mind plays in every aspect of your life? This includes your relationships, business, diet, health, and spiritual evolution. What you think about will materialize in your life. Your thoughts create your world. As you think, you become.

———————— ⟲⟳ ————————

Everything is a state of mind,
including your state of health.
If your thoughts are of health,
health will come to you.

———————— ⟲⟳ ————————

Your mind can be your greatest asset or your worst nightmare depending on how you care for it. I am saying "care" because, in one sense, the mind is like a child you must raise properly so that it can make the most out of life. In another sense, it is not unlike a powerful genie that will either work for you by granting your wishes or stalk you through demonic regions.

Perhaps you've tried to lose weight in the past. Perhaps you've tried to be healthier. Was it the "diet" that failed you or was it the way you were thinking? Perhaps you've made countless resolutions to be more cheerful or happier. Did your mind cooperate? It may be that negative thoughts have caused you to make choices that undermine your health. Before you ever take the step to exercise, don't you first make a mental decision to do so?

How often does your mind turn against you? You want to be healthy. You want to lose weight. You want to make your diet better. And yet, you find yourself going against your own goal. Perhaps you're too hungry to make sure what you eat is in line with your desire to improve your diet. That's what your mind tells you. Or maybe it tells you to "start tomorrow." Perhaps you think there's so much poison in the food supply, there's no sense trying—another thought that is not serving you.

MARILYN

As a little child, I was considered the "happy" one in my family. Huge dimples graced my cheeks, like those of my maternal grandmother, Ida, and, to hear the stories my relatives told, I, like Ida, was full of love, laughter, and good cheer. My grandparents, uncles, and aunts would use the Yiddish term of endearment "punim" whenever they referred to my little face with oversized dimples, and friends of the family always took me on their knees.

In the neighborhood, the older children played with me as if I were their doll. Apparently, in the years before I can remember, I would sit on the front stoop of our house, waiting for passersby, a child so small voicing such a melodic, friendly, tiny-voiced "HI!" that they would invariably be surprised. As I look at old family photo albums, I recognize in my face the pure essence of innocent joy that we each bring with us when we enter the world.

Ah, how do we lose it? What subtle battering, what series of pitfalls, deal the fatal blow to the love and happiness we know as children? By the time I had reached midlife, family photos record a totally opposite state of being. My adult life, in spite of tremendous effort, had so disappointed my dreams. Seeking love, I could only seem to uncover denial. Professional success and celebrity notwithstanding, I was living in a private world of pain and disillusion.

And how I chastised myself for the failure of my first marriage and the traumas divorce had brought to my two older children. From the moment I knew I would one day be a mother, it had been my only intention to give to my children all the security that I had been given as a child. Divorce was a stain of failure I could not wash from my psyche.

With determination and resolve that such failure could never again happen in my life, I struggled to make a secure and happy home in my second marriage. In spite of dire inner warnings and deep wounds that were inflicted on myself and my children, practically from the moment I took the vow, I resolved to turn the situation around and make it work. Despite the continuous psychological abuse, the media and fans demanded only a happy side. How it pained me, year after year, to see my children growing older in an atmosphere of stress, rather than one of love, with only the outward trappings of a stable home. The pressures I put on myself to try to offset the unhealthful environment of my marriage were literally draining my life force.

In 1980, I turned for assistance to Eastern spiritual study and meditation, seeking within solutions to the problems in my life. I would awaken at four A.M. and meditate until six. Almost every day, I would go to an ashram near my home and chant the hour-long morning prayer, seeking God's help. In the evening, I would return to the ashram as often as possible for chanting and meditation.

For years I did this, praying that somehow the sad environment in which I was living would lift, somehow heal, somehow become the bright and cheerful echo of my early childhood experience. I gave with all my heart to bring that dream to fruition. The task demanded every ounce of my energy and more.

I dreaded the idea that the only solution was another painful divorce and continued upheaval in my life. In spite of all my efforts spiritually, in spite of all the physical, mental, and emotional dedication I brought into the life I had chosen, I felt stuck and, because of this, on a very deep level I was filled with frustration at what had happened in my marriage, disappointment and fear that it might never end.

Then, in 1992, I heard about Dr. Schnell's weekend intensives, the East Meets West Hypno-Meditation Experience. I attended the first and immediately embraced MINDTONICS. When I first heard Dr. Schnell say, "You are living in a prison of your own making" to the group of participants, his words went straight to my heart. When he spoke of thoughts as those *"keys" that open the door to happiness or keep it solidly locked against us, a crack in my armor of self-destruction appeared.*

Suddenly I understood that I had the power to see my world the way I wanted to see it. I could create a different life for myself. These may be basic concepts, but to those who are struggling against all odds, or are drowning in their uncertainties, they can be life preservers at the right time. Happily, it was my moment. I began to realize that I had the power to think any thought I chose, and if I needed to change my life, that change would begin with my thinking.

MINDTONICS gave me a new picture. Once I began to put it into practice, I never needed to dwell in the regions of personal disempowerment, self-invalidation (or insidious invalidation coming from another), fear, loneliness, and despair. Thoughts of anger, inadequacy, and lack might drift across my mind, but the hold they could take in the mental "garden" I was cultivating was more and more temporary. I recognized them immediately as weeds, and pulled them just as quickly to make room for the healthy mental seeds I was constantly planting.

I learned TAKE FIVE!—a basic "attitude of gratitude" that completely changed my mental state from the "cup half empty" to "my cup runneth over." That one process ensured that I never again started my day without setting my own personal mental program, which included the cheerful disposition inherent in my nature. I experienced firsthand the truth that if I didn't program myself for happiness and success, external circumstances might easily program me for misery and gloom. And finally, I learned SELF-TALK, a way of setting the tone for my day every time I looked in the mirror.

These were just two aspects of MINDTONICS I was able to use to bring myself to a whole new level of existence. I became so excited about my ability to shape my world mentally, I began to recognize that missing component in practically everyone I knew. MINDTONICS brought me the ability to take a very important, very necessary, evolutionary step.

Mental Overload

At no time in human history have the minds of our species been subjected to such an enormous and continuous glut of information. This overconsumption of mental input causes MENTAL INDIGESTION—one of the main causes of the toxic society in which we live. Mental indigestion leads to classic thoughts like:

"I can't take any more."

"This is more than I can handle."

"I'm on overload."

Such thoughts may lead to behaviors such as eating a quart of ice cream or a whole box of candy or drinking the whole bottle of wine in order to "feel better." They may be among the prime reasons for reaching for a cigarette. They can also lead to giving up your determination to be healthy.

Socrates, the first Western guru, has held a respectful place in history as one of our greatest philosophers because of the advice he gave us on how to use our minds to enhance our lives. In fact, some people maintain that it was his wife, Xanthippe, who was the true source of his wisdom.

Be that as it may, we learn from them: "The life which is unexamined is not worth living." In other words, we must think about how we are living. If Socrates and Xanthippe were alive today, perhaps they would tell us that "the quality of our lives will improve when we change the quality of our thoughts."

Take the First Step to Spiritual Health

It's easy to say we should stop, examine our lives, and take charge of our thoughts, but it is, in fact, quite difficult to do. First of all, the mental overconsumption from too much input and the resulting mental indigestion make it very difficult to use the mind in a constructive way. In addition, we don't know how, because in our culture we are not instructed in the "how-to" of the mind.

From kindergarten through college, we treat our brains as information-collection bins, stuffing them with all manner of useless facts and figures. The most useful information—how the mind works, how to use it—is never taught. This is not unlike being given the keys to a car without any driving instruction. The consequences to our national health have been disastrous. For one thing, we don't know how to keep inevitable worry or frustration in check. One result has been an increase in suicide, particularly in teens, in the last twenty-five years. And just about every medical condition we're experiencing, from obesity to high blood pressure, has a strong mental component.

Think about it: How can you make clear, helpful choices in diet and exercise if you feel as if you're "flying off the handle," or "going off the deep end," if you continuously feel as if you will "snap" or "fall apart," or if you experience any of the numerous states that these expressions could describe? Can we let the problem become worse?

Let's face it, in adult life most Americans have few ideas about how to make the mind function to achieve health, happiness, and peace in their lives. To this basic flaw in our development we can trace the epidemic of disease, violence, gang killings, wife beating, child abuse, broken families, and depression in our country.

MINDTONICS

This MINDTONICS program is the "Operator's Manual" for your mind. It is based in active thinking. Active thinking is self-directed. Passive thinking is totally stimulated by outside or external influences.

Most important, we recommend that you use this MIND-TONICS program for at least thirty days. We have proven to ourselves that it takes at least that length of time to experience the beneficial effects of this new lifestyle.

Before Every Action, There Is a Thought

This is a scientifically proven fact. Have any of the following ever been part of your inner dialogue?

▶ "I can't help it, everyone in my family is overweight." *(As you help yourself to a pint of Ben and Jerry's.)*

▶ "Depression is normal nowadays." *(As you pop a pill.)*

▶ "Nobody cares about me anyway." *(As you pour yourself another drink.)*

▶ "I'm not as young as I used to be." *(As you take the elevator.)*

▶ "I can't cope with all the pressure." *(As you light another cigarette.)*

▶ "I don't have enough energy to eat right and exercise, not with my schedule." *(As you flop on the couch with a beer and a bag of chips.)*

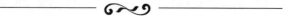

*Until you change your thinking,
you're not going to change your reality.*

It doesn't matter what kind of food or drug you put into your body, if you don't start looking at your thoughts and changing them from self-destructive to self-constructive, you're never going to achieve your goals of health and happiness. Are you ready to learn how to do this?

The first step is to tune in, examine your thoughts, and see if they're serving you. If they're not, change them.

Your Personal Channel

Every day, unless you create a positive program for yourself, your mind is programmed by outside influences. For example, when bad weather makes you feel blue, you can say:

"I can't take one more snowstorm."

"Rain again? If I don't see the sun soon, I think I'll go crazy."

Or, you can say, "The weather does not determine my happiness."

A snide remark from a coworker can completely ruin your week. If your boss ignores you, you may have trouble falling asleep that night, wondering what you've done wrong. Financial worries can force you to completely miss the joy on your child's face as he or she shares a success at school. All these situations, and many others, will determine your mental program UNLESS you take charge and spend a few minutes each day programming yourself.

Put it in perspective! Your mind is a tool, a mental servant, just as your hands and your legs are useful body tools. You wouldn't want your legs or your hands operating out of control, would you? So why should you allow your mind to always have its way? Just because your mind tunes into a certain thought, a negative "radio wave" passing through, doesn't for a moment mean that's the only thought worth thinking.

Pretend for a minute that your mind is like a television in your head that runs programs and changes channels all day long automatically. You can decide that it is time for you to pick up the controls. Instead of watching the "They Hurt Me, They're to Blame" or "Why I'm Doomed to Fail" soap operas, you can begin to air programs on your "Mind Network" that are all about your ability, happiness, and success. You can inject your mental program with elements of faith, trust, and gratitude that will connect you to the peaceful, harmonious, and loving state of your Soul. Happiness is the natural state of the Soul.

Like Learning to Ride a Bike

This exciting, yet troubled, era indicates that it's time to take charge, individually and collectively, and align ourselves with the higher goal of attaining spiritual peace and the power and happiness it brings.

We learn new skills by practicing them daily. As a child you learned to walk, ride a bike, or read—little by little. Everything you accomplished took practice. Adult learning is no different. Little by little, you can learn to completely manage your thoughts. Remember the Spanish proverb *"Poco a poco, se va lejos"* ("Little by little, one goes far").

As you use these simple exercises every day, they will be recorded over time in your storehouse of mental programs and, little by little, will begin to replace some of the destructive, negative programs your mind is now running automatically.

The goal is to *cleanse* the mind and throw out obsolete and harmful programs that don't serve your dreams. It is time to "dust away" the mental clutter that isn't helping you to reach the indwelling spirit and a new state of strength, happiness, and health.

Here's the key. Happy thoughts cleanse away sad ones. (And there's always something you can be happy about!) Confident thoughts cleanse away feelings of failure. Thoughts of approval cleanse away the programs of personal unworthiness and low self-esteem you have acquired. Now, let's begin.

Take Five

The great American philosopher Henry David Thoreau always took the first five minutes upon awakening to think about what was *right* in his life. This is how he set the tone for the rest of his day. We do the same, and we want you to try it as well.

What is good? What is working in your life? What can you be happy about? Count the small blessings you tend to take for granted and the large ones you sometimes neglect to appreciate. Do you have a roof over your head? A car? A job? Children? Food to eat?

Search your mind. If you don't do this, you can drag yourself out of bed in a negative frame of mind—and drag yourself through a day that gets worse with each passing hour—just because you allowed your day to start in a robotic, automatic way. A good way to end TAKE FIVE! is with a great, big, audible THANK YOU! for all that is right in your universe.

The gratitude that you express first thing in the morning will set your mood for your entire day. If you find yourself experiencing lack, even for a moment, you'll reconnect to the abundance you acknowledged and you'll change your thought.

Self-Talk

Once you've completed TAKE FIVE! have a brief conversation with yourself before you interact with others. Go to a mirror. *Talk to yourself!* Say out loud, "This will be a great day!" Mean what you say when you add, "Challenges are my opportunities to remain strong and upbeat."

Personalize your program, and repeat it several times. Look at yourself carefully while you say it. Believe it. Program love, happiness, success, and excitement. (If you don't, you risk being programmed by others for anger, sadness, failure, or boredom.)

Try new words or sentences to cleanse your habitual thought stream. Use the words *dynamic, exciting, fabulous, terrific, marvelous, exhilarating* in your SELF-TALK. Or repeat a sentence you might not even say, such as: *"I'm going to have the time of my life today. This is the best day of my life."*

All day long, the echoes of your SELF-TALK will reverberate and keep you on track. If you fall into the old habit of indulging a negative program, you'll hear it and pull yourself right out of it.

Dr. Norman Vincent Peale tells us, "Studies by psychologists, including Richard Lazarus and Shelly Taylor of the University of California, and Jonathan Brown at Southern Methodist University, point out that sunny optimism, or in their words, 'positive illusions' (in which people remember their strong points and successes more than their weaknesses and failures), promotes a sense of well-being, happiness, and the capacity for good, productive work. Those who think in the opposite, it seems, often tend toward mental problems, such as depression."[1]

Act Up!

We all played "make believe" as children. This is something we *know* how to do. The strategies we used as children to feel our power, like when we pretended to be Zorro or the Queen of England, are no less relevant now that we are adults.

Pretend? How can that help? Isn't that just creating a false persona? Remember William James, the professor of philosophy at Harvard University? He taught us that all behavior follows our thoughts. Therefore, if you want to be enthusiastic, you've got to *act* enthusiastic. If you want to be happy, start by *acting* happy.

---

[1]Norman Vincent Peale. *The Power of Positive Living*. New York: Ballantine Books, 1990, pp. 29–30.

We don't know about you, but we want to be fired up about life. We know for us, just as you can take the weight off your body, you can take the depression out of your mind. Let's not kid ourselves. ACTING UP is just like putting our best foot forward. If you can put a smile on your face for an interview for a new job, you can smile at your family, friends, and colleagues at the end of the day.

Spend the day acting upbeat, until that feeling is firmly rooted. Look at difficult moments as challenges, not disasters. Keeping things in a positive perspective will allow you to enjoy life much more. As you pretend your programming is real, it becomes real. It becomes who you are. It's like acclimating yourself to a new job. You have to give it that extra effort at first, and soon it's comfortable and you feel it's truly yours.

Actors and actresses can learn a new part. They can play tragic figures, saints, and criminals, all by just rehearsing the role until they have it down. "All the world's a stage" and you're learning your new part.

Leap Out of Your Rut!

You're ready to take control of yourself. If the rut you're in had worked for you, you wouldn't be worried about your health or weight and you wouldn't be wishing for a change.

Take a moment to do the following exercise: Stand up, slump your body, look down, wrinkle your brow, and frown. Connect to how this posture feels. Now, lift your head, look up to the sky, straighten your shoulders. Take a deep breath, hold it, slowly exhale, and SMILE! How does that feel? If you work on your posture, holding yourself erect, if you breathe and smile, it's hard to have a negative thought or run a pessimistic program.

Lynn Andrews, author of *Medicine Woman*, says, "The life force pours out of you through the holes you create in your life through addiction. The worst are emotional addictions, such as addiction to sadness, to chaos, to a feeling that we are not good enough."

This MINDTONIC is particularly relevant for those who wish to break a negative habit, such as smoking or sugar binge-ing. Normally, if you are a smoker, you will use one hand or the other to lift a cigarette to your lips. Characteristically, a certain posture will go along with the mind-set. "It's time to indulge myself and have a cigarette."

As soon as you are aware of the need to smoke, here are the steps to take:

▶ First, immediately stand up. Plant your feet firmly on the ground in a good, strong posture.

▶ As you're standing straight, look up, feeling strong and confident.

▶ Exhale, clear your lungs, take charge.

▶ If you are right-handed, lift your left hand, as if it held a cigarette, to your lips.

▶ Breathe in consciously, inhale a deep satisfying lungful of fresh air, hold it for about five seconds, and then slowly exhale.

▶ Feel your strength as you mentally say to yourself, "I'm a nonsmoker. I'm in control here. I have incredible will-power."

Use this same technique when you have a sugar craving. One of the first signs of dehydration is a sensation of hunger. Reach for a glass of water with the hand opposite the one you would use to reach for a donut. Use the water to flush, instead of clog, your body. Stand tall. Act tall. Be tall. Affirm the strength and health you are building in your body. Take a brief walk with confident strides.

You are in charge of your mind and your body. And you want to live healthfully. Remember, every action is preceded by a thought. Your addictions end when you change your thoughts.

Journal Work

This is the simplest of exercises and a concrete way to become more familiar with and grounded in your strengths, your goodness, and the side of you that you wish to reinforce. Keep a small spiral notebook with you, and whenever you think about a quality in yourself that you admire or approve of, jot it down.

What do you like about yourself? Do you have great handwriting, keep your desk organized, sew well? Do you tuck your children in at night, help others who are in need? Do you continuously try to read to expand your mind, go regularly for a haircut, call your parents once a week? Do you support others to reach their health goals? Remind yourself of the big things and the little things.

Please avoid a tendency to ignore or underestimate this exercise! Some of us are so busy thinking about what's wrong with us that we never even begin to notice our good qualities. What makes you feel better? An insult or a compliment? Actively listing all that is right about you will help you change your mental program and picture about yourself.

Don't Get Stuck Below Neutral

There are three basic possibilities for your emotional state:

1. **Positive:** constructive, cheerful, warm, optimistic, forgiving, enthusiastic, joyful, or happy.

2. **Neutral:** Nonemoting, productive, observant, calm, clear, or relaxed.

3. **Negative:** depressed, helpless, discouraged, miserable, tense, pessimistic, angry, fearful, or judgmental.

Ideally, because positive or neutral emotions are the most health-generating, you would wish to stay in the upper two states and keep yourself from getting stuck in neutral.

According to Dr. Martin Seligman, "Researchers looking at the immune systems of helpless rats found that the experience of inescapable shock weakens the immune system. T-cells from the blood of rats that become helpless no longer multiply rapidly when they come across the specific invaders they are supposed to destroy. These findings show that learned helplessness doesn't just affect behavior; it also reaches down to the cellular level and makes the immune system more passive.

"So the first way in which optimism might affect your health . . . is by preventing helplessness and thereby keeping immune defenses feistier. Optimism will also help you stick to a health regimen. Consider a pessimistic person who believes that sickness is permanent, pervasive and personal. 'Nothing I do matters,' he believes, 'so why do anything?' Such a person is less likely to give up smoking . . . diet . . . exercise."

Dr. Seligman proves his point in his report on a thirty-five-year-long study of one hundred Harvard graduates. It was discovered that pessimists were less likely than optimists to give up smoking and more likely to suffer illness.[2]

If you need more proof of the effect of your emotional state on your health, note that in a pioneering British study, sixty-nine women with breast cancer were followed for five years. Those who survived tended to have a fighting spirit, whereas those who died or suffered relapses tended to respond with helplessness or acceptance.[3]

[2]Martin Seligman. *Learned Optimism.* New York: Simon and Schuster, 1990, pp. 172–73.
[3]Ibid., p. 175.

▼ Even at Our Darkest Moments . . .

Great insights into the control and appropriate use of the mind come from the worst nightmare on earth—the concentration camp. Dr. Victor Frankel, author of *Man's Search for Meaning*, garnered fantastic revelations about the mind during his imprisonment in a Nazi concentration camp.

Frankel observed that those prisoners who used their minds to look for meaning instead of hopelessness withstood the hardships much better and were better able to put their lives together after the ordeal.

Corrie Ten Boom, a Christian author, also noted that those prisoners who prayed and had hope for the best fared better in the concentration camps. If the use of the mind can make such a powerful difference in a concentration camp, then imagine how this resource can be of benefit in your life.

▲

William James, the famous Harvard psychologist, stated that we use only 10 percent of our brains. As a result, most of the time we are operating in an automatic, habitual state of unconsciousness. George Gurdjieff, the Russian philosopher, believed that most people live their entire lives in a zombielike state he called "sleep." What about you? Are you on automatic pilot, asleep at the wheel?

▼

**The Seventh Principle
of Natural Health and Weight Loss**

To ensure health and happiness, make a regular effort, especially first thing in the morning, to mentally set the tone for the day.

▲

At the moment probably not, for Gurdjieff also taught that to learn of this "sleep" condition could be enough to awaken you, at least momentarily. But it takes effort to stay awake. He named this "waking up" process "self-remembering."

Reading these words can help you awaken and regain control of your mind temporarily, but the tendency to be "asleep" is so strong that it takes the daily use of mental exercises such as MINDTONICS to sustain the "awakened" condition. The mind is tricky. More than any other part of you the mind refuses to be disciplined. It takes perseverance and self-discipline to win the battle against laziness and defeat.

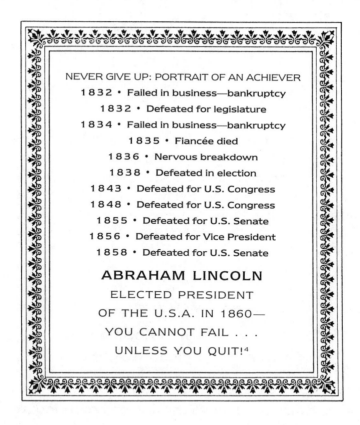

NEVER GIVE UP: PORTRAIT OF AN ACHIEVER
1832 • Failed in business—bankruptcy
1832 • Defeated for legislature
1834 • Failed in business—bankruptcy
1835 • Fiancée died
1836 • Nervous breakdown
1838 • Defeated in election
1843 • Defeated for U.S. Congress
1848 • Defeated for U.S. Congress
1855 • Defeated for U.S. Senate
1856 • Defeated for Vice President
1858 • Defeated for U.S. Senate

ABRAHAM LINCOLN

ELECTED PRESIDENT

OF THE U.S.A. IN 1860—

YOU CANNOT FAIL . . .

UNLESS YOU QUIT![4]

---

[4]*Journal of Financial Freedom*, "LIFEMONEYSUCCESS." February 1996, p. 5.

It's not just in the reading or the knowing, but in the *daily application* that these simple MINDTONICS begin to bear their fruit. We heartily encourage you to use them for thirty days. Using them can truly change your life. These are just a few to get you started.

We use them and many more every day of our lives to keep ourselves in the highest, most productive, happiest, and healthiest mental and emotional state. As you see a daily improvement in your health, as the weight drops off and your energy explodes, you'll see that MINDTONICS will have brought you to a new level of existence.

In a very short time, you will be a different person, shining your bright light on those around you, rather than a cloud of darkness. Once you have taken control of your mind, you begin to live in the state of celebration that human existence deserves.

If people tell you they've heard all of this before, and it simply can't be that easy, understand that you are listening to the voice of skepticism. But remember: Whatever we believe and expect will come to pass!

Historical MINDTONICS—coming from Buddha, Christ, Latin proverbs, and the Bible—echo this wisdom:

► As you sow, so shall you reap.

► What you focus on becomes your destiny.

► What you exhibit outwardly, you are inwardly.

► What you believe yourself to be, you are.

► Believe that you have it and you have it.

► All that we are is the result of what we have thought.

► The secret of success lies not without, but within, the thought of man.

These are timeless pearls of wisdom, articulated by the Great Teachers throughout the ages. To find your own pearls of wisdom and connect to your own Inner Teacher, to learn how to dive deep within yourself you can learn about . . .

11

▼

Hypno-Meditation: East Meets West

▼

*"Nothing should be omitted in an art
which interests the whole world,
one which may be beneficial to suffering humanity
and which does not risk human life or comfort."*
—HIPPOCRATES

In the East, meditation has been thoroughly developed; one could say that the East leads the world in this area. In the West, hypnosis has been thoroughly developed; one could say we're the masters in this field. The brand-new breakthrough for your health and well-being is the marriage of meditation and hypnosis that you will find in FITONICS. We call it Hypno-Meditation.

Hypnosis—It's Not What You Think

Hypnosis?

"Isn't that when someone on a stage in Las Vegas makes a volunteer from the audience bark like a dog?"

Okay, but that's not the kind of hypnosis we're talking about.

"Well, my friend used hypnosis to stop smoking."

Now you're getting warmer.

In fact, the American Medical Association shows a 78 percent success rate for smoking cessation utilizing hypnotherapy (hypnosis) as the treatment.[1] And this finding merely exposes the "tip of the iceberg." The application of hypnosis for healing purposes is probably the most exciting nonchemical, noninvasive, undersold, natural mental breakthrough in our era.

An Ancient Skill

Yet there's absolutely nothing new about hypnosis. Dr. Herbert Benson, author of *The Relaxation Response,*[2] a bestselling book in the 1970s, cites numerous historical "religious practices" that brought participants to "altered states of consciousness."

Such methods date back to the Assyrio-Babylonian physician-priests, the Egyptian soothsayers, and ancient Hebrew rabbis. The latter used magical rites, incantations, and meditation—accompanied by chanting, breathing exercises, and fixation on letters in the Jewish alphabet that spelled *God*—in ritualistic practices that were similar to autohypnosis and brought about a state of euphoria known as *kavanah*.[3]

According to two experts on hypnosis, Dr. William Kroger and Dr. William Fezler, this hypnotic state of *kavanah* in its "methodical meditation, breathing exercises, and ecstasy states [is] similar to the practices of Yoga, Zen Buddhism, Hinduism, Shintoism, Sufism, and Christian meditation."[4]

Early Chinese philosophers such as Lao-tzu, the founder of the religion of Taoism, believed that negative (Yin) forces

---

[1]The Atwood Institute, Course in Hypnotherapy, Phoenix, Ariz., 1995.
[2]Herbert Benson. *The Relaxation Response.* New York: Avon Books, 1975.
[3]William S. Kroger and William D. Fezler. *Hypnosis and Behavior Modification.* Philadelphia: Lippincott, 1976, p. 7.
[4]Ibid., p. 7.

caused disease that they were able to overcome by representing vivid images of positive (Yang) forces to the sick.

In ancient Greece, Hippocrates and Plato used hypnosislike methods to naturally treat mental disorders. The hundreds of Aesculapian healing temples found around 500 B.C. in Greece and throughout the Roman Empire all included a "dream healing" room, which was considered in that era to afford the best therapy for disease. After analyzing the patient's dreams, priests would induce a deep state of relaxation and use guided imagery and suggestion to alleviate the symptoms.

The literature of Zen and Tibetan Buddhism and Yoga abound as well with references to guided fantasies that were given to patients in a deeply relaxed state of contemplation.

A Modern Rediscovery

Franz Mesmer, the first Westerner to explore using the hypnotic state for healing, coined the word *mesmerism*. Like the Aesculapian priests, he would literally "brush away" symptoms of disease with the touch of his hand.

Although Mesmer laid the foundation for modern-day psychiatry with his theories of "animal magnetism," it was ironic that a luminary such as Benjamin Franklin, the discoverer of electricity, another form of magnetism, would investigate Mesmer's work and dismiss it as "all in the patient's head." Regretfully, Mesmer died in exile and in poverty.

"A commission was set up in 1784 by the Academie des Sciences to investigate Mesmer's animal magnetism cures; it concluded that 'magnetism without the imagination produces nothing.' Deslon, a member of the committee, stated, 'If the imagination is so effective, why do we not use it?'

"His question has been ignored for 200 years, as it is only recently that imagery technics are employed in psychiatry. This is surprising, as all religions control behavior by imagery conditioning."[5] It is more ironic still as we discover today that our belief in any treatment we embrace will determine whether or not that treatment will ultimately work for us.

The father of modern hypnosis is acknowledged as Dr. James Braid, who coined the term in 1889. But he was only one among many of the medical pioneers in hypnosis who were called charlatans by their colleagues (similarly to the Natural Health pioneers, whose work was rejected by traditional medical practitioners). For example, Braid's close friend and associate, the famous surgeon Dr. Esdaile, performed hundreds of major surgeries, including amputations, using hypnosis as the only anesthetic.

Esdaile was so ridiculed by "the scientific herd" that he died in shame and poverty. (During the same era in Europe, a Dr. Semmelweis was so hounded and ridiculed that he ended up in an insane asylum for beseeching his fellow surgeons to wash their hands after autopsies, before performing surgery, or when delivering a baby.)

Sigmund Freud, the father of modern psychotherapy, launched his practice with hypnosis, and his first book focused on the subject of hypnotherapy. But it was known that Freud was not good at using hypnotic techniques, and he abandoned them, keeping only the sofa, which was the original "hypnotic couch."

In 1955, the British Medical Association reported its approval of hypnosis, advising that all physicians and medical students receive fundamental training in the practice of hypnosis in their courses of study. Of course, this didn't take hold, because pharmaceuticals were easier to administer and made far more money. (Contrary to the teachings of Hippocrates, modern healers decided that it was easier and more profitable to drug a patient than to use an equally effective noninvasive form of therapy.)

---

[5]Ibid., p. 8.

In 1958, the American Medical Association recommended that "in view of our increasing knowledge, medical schools should include hypnosis in their curricula."[6] At this time, a very small percentage of medical schools offer a course of study in hypnotherapy, a number comparable to the small percentage that offer nutrition.

Hypnosis Is Real

Most often, today, hypnosis is used as the only anesthesia for surgical patients who are allergic to anesthetics. It is used to control blood flow, to hasten recovery, and to provide pain relief. In fact, studies done with people pretending to be hypnotized, along with those who are genuinely hypnotized, show that the pretenders always drop out of the experiment when it comes time to test for pain tolerance.

For example, a hypnotized patient can painlessly take a needle in the gum. One who is faking clearly feels the insertion. In double-blind studies to determine the validity of the hypnotic state, the experimenter works with two groups, only one of which has been hypnotized—the other is simply pretending. Temporary deafness is then suggested to both groups. When a gun is fired, pretenders flinch and jump. Those who are truly under hypnosis remain completely still.

Hypnosis is also used successfully for natural childbirth, to control nausea and vomiting in labor; for pain management in cancer treatment; for weight reduction and cessation of smoking; in psychiatric treatment for amnesia; to control the emotional causes of asthma; to stimulate regular menstruation and relieve menstrual cramping and tension; to augment breast size; for all psychosomatic disorders; for sexual dysfunction; to treat premature ejaculation and female infertility; for pediatric stuttering, tics, nail-biting, and bed-wetting; and in dentistry as an-

---

[6]Ibid., p. 9.

esthesia and to control salivation, the gag reflex, and pain. Hypnosis is extensively used in sports therapy, as well.

In FITONICS, you will find one of the most uniquely relevant applications for hypnosis—as an aide to meditation for attaining peace, balance, confidence, self-esteem, and happiness in your life.

Meditation? OM?

"I am familiar with the superstition
that self-realization is possible only in the
fourth stage of life, i.e., sannyasa (renunciation).
But it is a matter of common knowledge
that those who defer preparation
for this invaluable experience
until the last stage of life attain,
not self-realization but old age
amounting to a second and pitiable childhood,
living as a burden on this earth."
—LEO BUSCAGLIA, *PERSONHOOD*

"Isn't meditation something hippies used to do?"

"It's not for Christians, is it?"

"Well, my brother's doctor prescribed meditation to lower his blood pressure."

In fact, one of the best ways to lower blood pressure is to meditate. In *The Relaxation Response,* Dr. Herbert Benson noted that in a group of thirty-six participants who meditated regularly, there were measurable decreases in blood pressure that lasted as long as they meditated.[7]

Dr. Dean Ornish makes an indisputable case for the value of meditation in the pursuit of health. He tells us that some of its benefits are expanded awareness, increased concentration, a quieter mind, and the experience of transcendence, peace, joy,

[7]Benson. *The Relaxation Response,* p. 145.

and inner nourishment. Dr. Ornish specifically encourages a low-fat vegetarian diet for improved meditation.

Dr. Deepak Chopra tells us: "Science has discovered that the physiological state of meditators undergoes definite shifts toward more efficient functioning. Hundreds of individual findings showed lower respiration, reduced oxygen consumption, and decreased metabolic rate. In terms of aging, the most significant conclusion is that the hormonal imbalance associated with stress—and known to speed up the aging process—is reversed . . . long-term meditators can have a biological age between five and ten years younger than their chronological age."[8] Dr. Chopra is telling us that just as sleep is the ultimate rejuvenator, the lowered physiological activity brought about by meditation brings similar results.

Many Paths to Peace

There are many different styles of meditation, which originated in the East. The goal of Eastern meditation is to achieve what is described in various ways as Cosmic Consciousness, ultimate bliss, profound peace, God-realization, Enlightenment, *Samadhi*, awakening of *kundalini*, or Nirvana. All the world's great teachers have indicated that spiritual evolution comes from a consistent effort to achieve this higher state of being or consciousness; it is our ultimate destiny. As Jesus Christ said, "Know ye not that ye are gods?"

What we are missing in this country is a user-friendly meditative technique that will allow us—regardless of religion, creed, or race—to go deeply into these higher spiritual states. Swami Muktananda, one of the most famous meditation teachers who brought meditation from the East to the West, assured us: "Sleep belongs to all people of all religions—Muslim, Hindu, Christian, and Jew; in the same manner, so does meditation."

[8]*Ageless Body, Timeless Mind.* New York: Harmony Books, 1993, p. 32.

Still, many Westerners have been afraid to approach meditation for fear they'd have to accept some new religion—or worse, follow a guru. Many feel meditation will take too much time or be too difficult and uncomfortable. That can be true for many forms of meditation that come from the East.

Largely because of the Beatles' discovery of Maharishi Mahesh and his Transcendental Meditation (TM) movement in the early 1960s, millions of Westerners have dabbled in Eastern meditation styles over the past thirty years, hoping to attain the higher spiritual states, or to at least improve their lives in some manner. We are intimately familiar with their experiences because we are among them.

It goes something like this: You go to an ashram or other designated place where meditation is taught. You are given a mantra. Perhaps you are taught chants. You are instructed in breathing techniques. You are encouraged to sit and clear your mind. There is sometimes a special way to sit, usually cross-legged. (Only if your back is weak are you encouraged to lean against something. For how many Westerners would that not be necessary, conditioned as we are to sitting in chairs and driving in cars, unlike our Eastern sisters and brothers who deftly sit on the floor and walk or bike where they need to go?)

The result of all this, for the largest numbers of people, is nonetheless beneficial. Many meditators find themselves calmer, more able to concentrate, and less likely to feel overwhelmed by daily life. There are also those who reach a higher or deeper experience, but rarely is this consistent.

The problem with placing the goal of meditation on what Dr. Ornish calls the "transcendent state" is that many people, feeling this is the only reason to meditate, spend frustrating time allowing their minds to rant on and on, and after months or years of this type of meditation, they are probably not much further along than when they started. They are not even more relaxed from their efforts.

Many others attempt meditation for a brief interval and then let it go, feeling occasionally guilty that they didn't follow through. And then there is the vast number of people who feel the whole thing is far too Eastern for red-blooded Americans. All of us need to put meditation in perspective and tap into a practical way to apply it to our lives.

Why Would You Want to Seek Cosmic Consciousness in the First Place?

The answer is a simple one, and yet it is not often articulated. First of all, it is from this higher state of awareness that our best human emotions flow. Joy, ecstasy, peace, compassion, inspiration, forgiveness; states that bring real positive meaning and achievement to life are all aspects of Cosmic Consciousness.

When we become rooted in the perspective, objectivity, and clarity of that state, we are able to do the best problem solving. It's well-known that famous inventors such as Thomas Edison and Henry Ford spent time alone in their studies to achieve the meditative state that would bring on inspiration. Every religion says that, in some form or other, our final destiny is to merge with the Universal Creative Principle. This is how we transcend all pain, discomfort, jealousy, envy, hatred, distrust, and bigotry while manifesting abundance, love, prosperity, tranquility, oneness, and charity.

If we look at history, our greatest leaders, male and female, have been those who embodied these qualities. Among these leaders are saints, philosophers, and the founders of the world's religions—the Mother Teresas, Martin Luther Kings, Martin Bubers, and Dalai Lamas.

▼
DR. SCHNELL TEACHES WHAT HE KNOWS BEST

My passion for Cosmic Consciousness began with my experience in the crib when I identified myself as the Light surrounding my body. I can to this day remember watching my grandmother carrying my infant twin brother down the hallway. I was floating above all of it, looking down, watching them and my body, there below me in the crib, from a field of Light.

Now, I know you're probably shaking your head, wondering, "What is this guy talking about?" Being in the Light is a *real, genuine* phenomenon, attainable by all.

My first experience as a spiritual teacher came at age four, when, in a state of eureka, I approached my playmate, four-year-old Charlie Foster, to inform him as he played horseshoes of a metaphysical insight. It had come to me that spring day in the Arizona desert, coinciding with my second experience of the Light.

"Charlie," I said breathlessly, full of wonder and excitement, as I stood in the shade of the house and squinted out into the blazing sun. I was digging my toes into the cool dirt, waiting for him to look at me.

"Charlie!" I insisted. "You are not your body! You are not your mind!"

Just as you can sit right now, observe your body, and hear your mind think, I realized then—and it was a great revelation to my young self—that I was not my mind, but rather "I" was the witness to my mind. I felt really good about the idea, very comfortable with it. Furthermore, I realized that my "I" and Charlie's "I" were one and the same, tiny "chips" off the cosmic "block."

Charlie received this news in a rather amusing fashion. He pulled the horseshoe stake out of the ground and bopped my brother Everett squarely on the head. My career as a spiritual teacher was off to a screaming start.

Around that same time, I was hiking in the long shadow cast by my six-foot-three father in the vicinity of Locomotive Mountain in the Southern Sonoran Desert when I was suddenly immersed for the third time, as if from the inside out, in a field of radiant, pure white Light. That experience and all the others of my early years have never left me. They are as clear today as they were nearly four decades ago.

I believe they led me to determine, at age seven, after my reading of Parmahansa Yogananda's exquisite spiritual journey in *Autobiography of a Yogi*, that I might one day be one of the spiritual teachers pictured on the many pages of photographs. With that inner commitment at such a young age, I began my years as a student of meditation.

From age seven to age twelve, and before I was old enough to be a certified member of the Self-Realization Fellowship, I diligently pursued the course of training through my father's weekly lessons. In the evening, when all my friends were watching *Gunsmoke* and *What's My Line?* on their black-and-white TVs, I would study the spiritual lessons. Late at night, while the rest of the family was sleeping, I would sit up in my bunk and meditate. My consistent study, identification with the masters, and practice gave me the ability to dive deep within, and on occasion I would there encounter inner visions.

After reading that yogis have such self-control they can regulate their heartbeats—in fact, on occasion stop and then restart them[9]—one afternoon in meditation, using a specific technique from Self-Realization Fellowship designed to accomplish that very goal, I clearly brought my own heartbeat to a stop for at least five minutes, until my stepmother came unexpectedly into my room, slamming the door, shouting, "Donald, get out of that trance!"

Poor Mom, a preteen yogic son in a copper-mining town in the 1960s was a little more than she had bargained for. If I had been older, I probably would have had a heart attack at that moment from the shock of going from total stillness and tranquility to the sudden jump start to everyday reality, and if she had known what I was actually doing, *she* would have had a heart attack.

My father was the only white child raised on the Tohono O'odham Indian Reservation in Arizona, which gave him the basic compulsion to be closer to God and Nature. Although underage, at age twelve, I began to study the lessons he was receiving from the Rosicrucian Order, the acknowledged oldest spiritual society in the world, older than Freemasonry, which traces its roots to ancient Egypt. At the same time, I developed a passion for the study of hypnosis, and when books on that subject were denied to me at the public library because they were not in the children's section, my teacher, Mrs. Leonard, checked them out for me.

At age eighteen, I began twelve years of formal training with weekly spiritual lessons from the Rosicrucians, reaching the level of Adept, and today I am in the higher degrees of that Order. I had the good fortune, at age nineteen, of enrolling in a seventeen-year program of spiritual study with Dr. Hugh Greer Carruthers, an Oxford scholar and surgeon who became a Tibetan lama during a seventeen-year sojourn in a monastery in Tibet.

The most important learning I imbibed from Dr. Carruthers was that the thoughts we think create our lives. He gave me the gift of the ages—not just

---

[9]This example of mental control, considered impossible by traditional medicine, was demonstrated to medical doctors by Swami Rama at the Menninger Clinic in Topeka, Kansas, in the 1970s.

the concept, but the actual power over my mind. In my twenties, I was accepted into the Martinist Order, an esoteric philosophical order that focuses on understanding the world's ancient religious principles; the Order was founded in the 1800s by the renowned French philanthropist and mystic Jean Claude Martin.

At one point I met Dr. Ramurti Mishra, an Indian doctor at New York's Bellevue Hospital, who was a psychiatrist, a surgeon, and a master of Oriental languages. He was also a swami, and he founded the first ashram in the United States, Ananda Ashram in upstate New York. Dr. Mishra also demonstrated the powers of the focused mind at week-long trainings I attended. I devoured all of Dr. Mishra's writings. His *Fundamentals of Yoga* became one of my most important references.

In the late 1970s, I enrolled in the Siddha Yoga Teachers Training under Swami Muktananda, and shortly after that I became the only civilian (non-swami) to run one of the four Siddha Yoga Dham Ashrams in the United States. For the next five years, I taught this style of meditation.

It was at around this time that I began my extended pilgrimages to India, studying under various renowned and lesser-known spiritual teachers. Between two trips, I connected with the late Dr. Jack Hislop, the founder of the American TM movement and the American movement under Sathya Sai Baba. Soon after I corresponded with Dr. Samuel Sandweiss, a psychiatrist at the University of San Diego and author of the book *The Holy Man and the Psychiatrist*, I was compelled to return to India, believing that Sai Baba was worthy of a firsthand experience.

In total, I spent nearly two years at the ashrams of Sathya Sai Baba, eight hours a day, under a merciless cloudless sky, sitting cross-legged on the dirt with hundreds of other people, meditating and waiting for interaction with the master. Those experiences, known in spiritual work as *tapasya*,[10] fully immersed me in the concept of guru and avatar.[11]

I witnessed hundreds of miracles at the hand of the holy man. To me, they were clear demonstrations of Sai Baba's love, his focused mind, his spiritual consciousness, and our evolution toward that consciousness within ourselves. There were many people at the ashram who had brought their illness to Sai Baba. One was a young paraplegic child, age twelve, brought by his father to sit day after day in his wheelchair, with unevenly focused eyes, lax jaw, saliva running down his chin and neck, in the scalding Indian summer. One day, after several weeks, completely and miraculously healed

---

[10]"Undergoing hardship for the sake of spiritual growth."
[11]Spiritual leader for the world.

by Sai Baba, he *charged* into me, like an ordinary child who wasn't paying attention, as I turned a corner with an ice-cream cone in my hand. His father, in a state of euphoria, was huffing and puffing to keep up with his son, who was running to join the line for ice cream. . . .

In the search for spiritual growth, we've all heard stories of the miraculous. We, ourselves, have witnessed and experienced countless examples ranging from levitation and firewalking to the rare materializations phenomenon. What we have learned from our spiritual journey is that the mind is an untapped resource that can bring us to a far greater potential than we can ever imagine—if only we apply ourselves.

There are many ways other than spiritual miracles to show mastery over the mind and make a difference on the planet. Mother Teresa's selfless giving is a lofty modern-day example. What are great expressions of art or music, if not manifestations of mental mastery and contributions to human happiness? What of the teacher in today's classroom who labors for low wages under frequently frustrating conditions, day after day, to materialize in children the ability to read, write, and live together in harmony? Look at the ballerina's mastery over her body. Or the mastery over personal emotional needs of a nurse, doing what others refuse to do for the sick in hospitals around our country.

For me, these are full-fledged spiritual manifestations. In my workshops and intensives, it is this well of power within each of us that I seek to uncover in others. It's important to me that people look inside themselves for the miracles within them; it's important that they find their own spiritual resources and begin to materialize in their actions the good within, which is found most easily in Hypno-Meditation.

▲

It's Time to Awaken

"A mighty flame followeth a tiny spark."
— D A N T E

The Yogis believe that every living being has potential spiritual energy that can be awakened. They call this the *kundalini*. When this energy awakens, one's spiritual evolution begins. According to the Buddhists, we step off the wheel, stop revolving in the same futile patterns, and begin an upward movement toward higher consciousness and greater reward in our lives. As this energy unfolds, we see more than before. We feel more than before. We are more aware.

It is said that the kundalini, or potential spiritual energy, lies dormant at the base of the spine. This is like being in possession of a match. If you wish to create a fire, it's not enough just to possess the match. Not enough just to read about it, think about it, hear about. You must take action. If you need fire, you have to strike the match.

If you seek spirituality in your life, it is the same. You have to take action. The right kind of action.

There are three states of consciousness. Everyone is familiar with at least two of them: the conscious mind and the subconscious mind. Dick Sutphen, a world-renowned metaphysician, defines conscious and subconscious mind:

"Conscious mind: will, reason, logic, and the five physical senses.

"Subconscious mind: the memory banks, containing all your past programming, including beliefs, habit patterns, emotional programming and the *Akashic* records[12] of all the lifetimes you have ever lived."[13]

---

[12]Memories of prior life experiences.
[13]Dick Sutphen. *Reinventing Yourself.* Malibu, Calif.: Valley of the Sun Publication, 1993, p. 155.

The third state, a spiritual state—the superconscious mind (higher self)—will not automatically be revealed. Dick Sutphen's definition:

"Superconscious mind: the creative force and psychic abilities, the collective awareness of mankind, plus unlimited unknown powers. When you attain a higher self level of consciousness, you have at your mental fingertips an awareness of your totality, and the collective totality of the energy *gestalt* we can call 'God.' We are all part of the collective unconscious—the greater body of mankind. Thus, we are all one."[14]

On occasion, people will stumble across the superconscious state by accident. For example, a person will hear a voice inside their head telling them not to board an airplane that later crashes. Or someone has an idea, and lo and behold, practically overnight the idea becomes a multimillion-dollar industry because others so needed it.

We use Hypno-Meditation successfully to bypass years of effort or random hit-or-miss strategies to access the superconscious mind for success in all aspects of our daily lives. This includes spiritual, mental, and physical well-being, and does not leave out the practical concerns of weight loss, breaking addictions, and improving health.

▼

The Eighth Principle
of Natural Health and Weight Loss

To find peace and harmony, take five to twenty minutes each day to deeply relax body and mind.

▲

---

[14]Ibid., p. 155.

Once you access superconsciousness, physical "limitations" seem to melt away. You have tapped into something greater than the physical: truly MIND OVER MATTER. It is the most powerful mind, the superconscious mind, the mind of the Soul.

Your Hypno-Meditation Session

The following instructions will be your guidelines for a twenty- to thirty-minute daily meditation session, designed to give you a deep and healing spiritual experience.

The time spent on meditation should be regarded as some of your most precious. It is your opportunity to connect with your soul and all of the good within you. Therefore, it is recommended that you:

▶ Choose a time when you are most relaxed, perhaps at night, before you go to sleep.

▶ If possible, choose a special room where you will not be disturbed for at least twenty minutes. Remember to turn off the phone.

▶ It helps to take a warm bath beforehand and to put on fresh clothes.

▶ Light a candle and incense, if you like, and play your favorite soft, tranquilizing music.

The attitude you bring to your session is crucial. A "prove-it-to-me" state of mind will only encourage you to remain in your ordinary waking consciousness. You will manifest the spiritual principle that what you believe manifests.

Begin by finding a comfortable easy chair or by lying down. Snuggle under a soft blanket and put some ear plugs on to shut the world out and help you concentrate on your breathing. For about two minutes, take deep, slow satisfying breaths. Go ahead, take one now. Inhale and then hold the breath for about five seconds, then slowly exhale through the mouth as you let go of all tensions in body and mind.

The breathing can make or break your session. Breathe with the conscious intention that you are pulling spiritual energy into your body with every breath you take. As you make a regular practice of meditating, you will learn that the key to getting the most out of this mental exercise is to BREATHE. Continuous, deep breathing calms and strengthens the mind.

There are five basic steps to Hypno-Meditation:

1. Relaxation

2. Deepening

3. Meditation

4. Constructive programming

5. Awakening

RELAXATION

During this phase, as you relax your body, it helps to visualize a warm washcloth twisted tightly between your hands. As you relax your muscles, visualize the washcloth untwisting and becoming loose and flat. Untwist your muscles in the same way.

Now is the time to sink back into your chair or bed. Feel the weight of your body as you allow yourself to become totally comfortable. Imagine a golden light, the warm light of the sun, coming down from the heavens. This golden light has the special power to relax you, warming and relaxing the scalp as it enters the top of your head. Create this sensation with the power of your own imagination. *Want* it to happen. *Expect* it to happen. *Allow* it to happen. *See* it happen. *Feel* it happen. Bring your awareness to your scalp. Remember the warm washcloth, untwisting, and imagine that all tension in your scalp is leaving. Say to yourself, "My scalp is relaxing." *Think* it, *feel* it, and *allow* it to happen.

Tell yourself that nothing from this moment on is going to interfere with your Hypno-Meditation. All outside sounds are now going to become a part of your relaxation. Each time you relax a body part, you are going to go deeper into the profound relaxation of Hypno-Meditation. You will use the washcloth symbol with each muscle group. Now concentrate on your forehead. You say to your forehead, ''Relax,'' as you picture the warm, soothing, washcloth untwisting.

Now, as your forehead relaxes, you may or may not notice a slight increase of tension around your eyebrows. Relax the eyebrows. If you haven't closed your eyes, now is a good time. Just tell yourself that as long as you keep your eyes closed you will remain in the Hypno-Meditative state. If you have the need to scratch at any time, you may move your left arm and hand without disturbing your depth. From this point forward you want to make yourself completely comfortable, and begin to remain still as a statue.

Tell yourself that with each passing minute you will now become more and more relaxed. In fact, with each and every breath you *will* become more and more relaxed from this moment on.

Now, shift your awareness to your eyes. Feel the relaxing power as you picture the golden light around your eyes. This light pushes out all darkness as it travels downward, pushing tensions out through imaginary openings in the fingers and toes. This inner sunlight calms and soothes every muscle, nerve, bone, and fiber of your body. Let the light come into your eyelids, relaxing the tiny muscles around the eyes. Now let it go deep into the eyes, and behind the eyes. Again picture the washcloth untwisting. Feel the relaxation now in your scalp, forehead, and eyes.

Relax your facial muscles, your jaw, and your lips. Relax the back of your throat. Tell yourself that your mouth will be moist, just enough to keep you perfectly comfortable. If you have to swallow, you can do so without thinking about it, and if you swallow, you will go deeper.

Relax your neck, the front, sides, and back. Visualize the relaxing power as it travels throughout your neck. It is the warm gentle, golden light of the sun. As it travels down your body you become more and more relaxed. The relaxing power now enters your shoulders, and you think, "My shoulders are relaxing." Picture the warm washcloth, and feel the muscles of your shoulders unwind even more as you go deeper and deeper into Hypno-Meditation.

Feel a wave of relaxation travel down your upper arms, elbows, forearms, and wrists. Suggest to each of these body parts that they relax. Allow your upper chest and back to relax. Tell your stomach to relax. Remember to picture the warm light of the sun in these areas, and use the symbol of the warm washcloth as well. You communicate with your subconscious through words and pictures.

Bring the warm, gentle light of the sun into your hips and thighs. Say to yourself, "My hips and thighs are now relaxing." *Believe* it, *expect* it, *want* it to happen, and *allow* it to happen. Picture the warm washcloth untwisting. Just let your tensions go. In the same fashion, relax your knees, lower legs, ankles.

Let the warm light of the sun flow into the feet as it sweeps all darkness out of your body. Let the light relax the bottoms of your feet, your insteps and toes. Now say to your entire body, *"Relax and let go."*

DEEPENING

You have relaxed the body. Now you begin to relax the mind in order to slide into the superconscious state.

Bring your awareness to the "third eye" region in the center of the forehead, just above the eyebrows. Anthony Robbins teaches in his seminars that when we look up, we are signaling the brain to put us into a more resourceful state. Jose Silva, founder of Silva Mind Control, popular in the 1970s, says that when we put our awareness into the space above the eyebrows, we will generate more alpha rhythms.

Researchers have long associated alpha rhythms with greater relaxation and a sense of well-being. Spiritual teachers in the East have taught that this process of looking up activates our spiritual willpower, as well as our spiritual vision. Biblically: "If thine eye is single, thy world is full of light."

While your gaze is focused upward, tell yourself that your body will continue to relax with each breath and each passing moment. Picture a large chalkboard in your mind. Imagine that you are standing in front of it with an eraser in one hand and red chalk in the other. Draw a circle on the board, and then write the number 25 within the circle. Carefully erase the number. Say to yourself, "As I count down to one, I will relax more deeply with each and every number. By the time I get to the number one, I will be in my superconscious mind."

Now continue to write each number in your circle. Pause for about two seconds, erase the number, and allow yourself to relax before going on to the next number. Don't worry if you don't make it all the way to 1. This is the process to allow your mind to let go and completely relax. Some people need only a few numbers for this to happen.

MEDITATION

The Quakers use the phrase "the still small voice within." The Yogis tell us we are in deep meditation when we stop the mental waves. Have you ever seen the moon reflected on the surface of a calm, placid lake? If the water is stirred up by the wind, the reflection disappears.

In a similar way, when your mind is calm, the superconscious mind can be experienced. As you proceed toward that goal, allow your mind to drift and float . . . drift and float. There is nothing you have to do, no one to satisfy. Just let go and allow the quietness to come in. Breathe gently, slowly, rhythmically. Continue to breathe gently, slowly, rhythmically while maintaining a gentle awareness within the third-eye region. Become very, very still. The Old Testament proclaims, "Be still, and know that I AM." This is your connection time to the Soul.

Allow as much time as you need. A minute in this space can seem like ten minutes, and on other occasions ten minutes may seem like a minute.

CONSTRUCTIVE PROGRAMMING

Out with the old; in with the new. This is the important few minutes you take to give your subconscious mind a new set of operating guidelines. Below are some sample suggestions:

▶ "I find I no longer have a craving for refined sugar and sugary products."

▶ "I can lose weight and I will do it by eating healthy, whole, and natural foods."

▶ "I have the inner strength to turn my back on cigarettes."

▶ "I now choose to stop drinking alcoholic beverages."

▶ "I experience life as divine harmony."

▶ "I am now open to all the beauty and happiness life has to offer."

▶ "I feel powerful and in control of my life."

▶ "My optimistic thinking creates a constructive life."

▶ "I have the willpower and ability to keep going."

▶ "I now call upon a higher power to keep me on the road to health."

This one step makes all the difference in your life. The power of old programs is very great. There is an old saying: "First you make your habits; then your habits make you."

Meditation notwithstanding, many seekers experience obstacles because they are ruled by their old habits. Procrastination, laziness, unwillingness to take responsibility, these continue to dominate and create pain. Constructive programming is such a powerful tool that when you are in the superconscious state, it can literally give your brain a brand-new set of operating instructions.

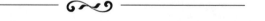

Before you start the process of Hypno-Meditation, choose an area of your life that you wish to improve.

Using the examples above, this is when you give suggestions to yourself that are particularly relevant to your personal situation, such as "I can pass up dessert at the next meal. I can get up tomorrow morning and exercise."

AWAKENING

To return from the state of Hypno-Meditation you will count yourself up by thinking:

- **"Number one.** I am returning. I am deciding to feel good and full of joy for life."

- **"Number two.** I am recalling the situation in my room. I am choosing to feel strong and healthy."

- **"Number three.** I am almost fully returned; I am aware of the temperature in the room."

- **"Number four.** I'm coming on up, and on the next count I will open my eyes and be wide awake. I feel fantastic!"

- **"Number five.** I am stretching and opening my eyes. I AM WIDE AWAKE!"

―――――――― ⟨∾⟩ ――――――――

What makes a fine pianist is not the sound of the scales each time he practices, but the consistent and constant practice. So it is with meditation. The experiences of meditation are wonderful . . . and sometimes just so-so. Remember, though, that it is not the experience per se, but the act of meditation which transforms us.

―――――――― ⟨∾⟩ ――――――――

Incorporating This Process into Your Life

If you awaken early in the morning, and there is time for you to do so, begin your day with your Hypno-Meditation session. If your mornings are too hectic, end your day with your session instead.[15] Once you have practiced for a while, you'll be able—during the day, at will—to reenter the superconscious state, feel the renewal therein, and slowly, over time, that state will override the conscious state of everyday living.

Life will take on the magical, blissful quality that comes from connecting to the Soul's upward movement through it, rather than the more limited up-and-down experience of body and mind. And you'll be able to support the divine flame you have ignited through . . .

―――――

[15]For those who are interested in guided Hypno-Meditation, the FITONICS HYPNO-MEDITATION tape is available at your local bookstore. Hypno-Meditation can be experienced in the FITONICS EXPERIENCE weekend workshops. For information, call 1-888-FITONIC.

PART THREE

THE DAILY EXERCISE
BREAKTHROUGH

12

▼

BODYTONICS

▼

"It takes twelve to twenty minutes at the advance level
and that's nothing compared to going to a gym,
which takes you the time to drive there,
time to work out, time to drive back . . .
I don't have that time.
Nobody does anymore, when you work.
I hated going to the gym.
I hated to make the effort. And I wouldn't do it.
And that's the whole thing.
BODYTONICS is different. It's so easy.
I like doing my legs. That's my favorite now,
so I concentrate on that area.
Then I go to my chest or back. I just break it up.
I always had a little definition,
but now my calf muscles are sticking out, and,
when I wear my little biker shorts,
people actually stop me and say,
'You know, you've got nice legs.'
I wish I could show you everything
that BODYTONICS have changed, but I can't.
But take my word for it.
Everything is getting a little perkier and a little uplifted."

—LYNN M.
(in an interview at the end of the FITONICS test)

Life Force

Life force can be seen. Look around and you will observe people
who glow. They have a natural, spontaneous smile, a sparkle in
their eyes, bounce and spring in their step. Children start out

with high levels of life force, and it is frequently said: "Children are closer to God." High levels of life force are associated with *youthfulness, energy,* and *spirituality.* President John F. Kennedy once said, "Physical fitness is not only one of the most important keys to a healthy body. It is the basis of dynamic and creative intellectual activity."

> "Exercise is good for your blood, writes *American Health.* Regular physical exercise seems to thin the blood by expanding the volume of plasma, the liquid portion of the blood. This ultimately means a reduced risk of blood clotting and, therefore, a lower stroke and heart attack risk."
>
> —"Fitness Health," *Muscular Development,* June 1996

Have you ever noticed that when a president takes office there's a noticeable radiance? There's a glow of victory. But as the demands of the office increase, the glow fades, and as it fades, popularity drops in the polls. The secret all successful people must learn is how to *recharge* the radiance that will ensure continued success.

Those in our society with the highest levels of life force are the achievers and the leaders. Opportunities just seem to drop into their laps. You wonder: "How is it they have all the luck—or is there a principle at work here?"

It is absolutely within your power to increase your life force. Dr. Gabriel Cousens says, "By consciously building the type of physical body that is able to be sensitive to, attract, conduct, nurture, and hold the higher spiritualizing energies, we become more capable of holding the full power of God's Light."[1] And what is God's light if not your very own LIFE FORCE, the glow of health?

On the other hand, you see people who waste their life force through alcohol, drugs, smoking, overeating of processed foods, and inactivity. They vibrate at low levels without fail, and seem to have barely enough energy to make it through the

---

[1]Gabriel Cousens. *Conscious Eating.* Santa Rosa, Calif.: Vision Books International, 1992, p. 149.

day. Their appearance is listless, lackluster, and they exude an air of exhaustion. Often they seem to want to sleep most of their lives away, almost as if they are too depleted to get out of bed. People functioning at a low level of vibration, from teenagers to senior citizens, are crowding doctors' offices, clinics, convalescent homes, and hospitals.

Life Flows to Life

It is a cruel truth that when life force is low, life doesn't send opportunities. Life flows to life. Is this intelligent energy going to give you a break if your body isn't able to cope with the extra surge? If you are low in energy, you probably can't even recognize when opportunity is knocking. Water seeks its own level. Opportunity will seek out those who have the energy to meet the demands. This is one of life's greatest secrets. If you want a better job, better opportunities, better health, a loving and attractive mate, then increase your life force!

However, for many of us, life seems to unfold in a predictable pattern. As we begin to lose our youth, a stream of pains and aches manifests as our reality. Constipation, insomnia, tired feet, stomach pain, high blood pressure, stiffness in the joints, headaches, and lethargy are all so much a part of daily life that they are taken for granted, much like the sun and the rain.

And what follows in their wake is a feeling of surrender and sadness, as if there is nothing that can be done. Except, of course, the taking of laxatives, antacids, blood pressure medication, pain pills, sleeping aids, alcohol, recreational drugs, and cigarettes. Yet, the President's Council on Physical Fitness has been telling us since the 1960s that most of our aches and pains are due to lack of exercise.

Like Attracts Like!
Health Attracts Health!

You have to play an *active* part. The person who says "Well, if you had my schedule, you wouldn't exercise either! After the day I put in, I can't do more than eat and crash in front of the television" is going to wake up ill. You've heard all the excuses, and so have we:

"Can't exercise, I have a bad knee."

"Not with my back."

"What good will it do? I'm fat, and I'll always be fat."

"I'm too old."

All these are affirmations that lead to premature aging and ill health. You have to take an active role in creating the conditions for good health to come your way.

You can add life force to your body by adding enzymes in the form of fresh vegetables, fruits, their juices, and enzyme supplements, but there is an equally important part to this equation. All food is metabolized by oxygen.

You can take in the best nourishment in the world, but if you are oxygen-starved, you are not going to burn up your food and use it as fuel. Instead, it will not metabolize completely, and you will suffer the consequences of internal pollution. Dr. Cousens says, "Poor oxygenation of the cells creates poor cellular oxidative metabolism and eventually cellular death."[2]

Jack LaLanne, the famous American fitness pioneer, tells us, "The harder you breathe, the more oxygen you take into your bloodstream and the faster you burn up fat. It's very similar to your fireplace; the more air you give your fire, the faster it burns. I like to think of us as combustion engines: the more we eat and the less we exercise, the slower the fat burns; but the

---

[2]Ibid., p. 145.

less we eat and the more we exercise, the faster we burn and lost the fat."[3]

Oxygen Starvation

Unfortunately, our overweight nation suffers from oxygen starvation. The situation is so bad that one medical doctor, Philip Rice, who worked his whole life with delinquent children, stated that 55 percent of delinquency in minors can be attributed to oxygen starvation.[4] How can he say that? Let's think about it for a moment.

Shallow breathers poison themselves by depriving their bodies of the adequate oxygen that keeps them clean. How does oxygen keep you clean? Walk into a dense forest, rich with the oxygen that is produced by all the trees and plants. Now lift a large rock that is lying in perpetual shade, under a bed of ferns. What do you see? Slime, bugs, the creepy-crawly matter that thrives in a dark, oxygen-deprived location. Fungal matter grows where oxygen is less plentiful. Bacteria and other microbes thrive there as well.

Your internal environment is no different from the condition we have just described. We spend days in air-conditioned or heated offices or homes, many of which have sealed windows. How can our bodies get the fresh air they need to feed adequate oxygen to our cells? Being sedentary causes inner stress. The organs of the body are not properly oxygenated without sufficient movement and exercise. When your body is oxygen-deprived, the result is a bloodstream that is forced to carry excess carbon dioxide and other poisonous gases and residues. Everything in your body is connected. If the blood is poisoned, the brain is poisoned, thoughts are poisoned, actions are destruc-

---

[3]Jack LaLanne. *Revitalize Your Life After Fifty.* Mamaroneck, N.Y.: Hastings House, 1995, p. 104.
    [4]Paul Bragg and Patricia Bragg. *Super Brain Breathing.* Santa Barbara, Calif.: Health Science, 1987, p. 5.

tive. If your blood is already burdened with poisonous wastes, how can it transport the necessary nutrients and the small amount of oxygen it does absorb to your cells?

Just as a room becomes stuffy and unbearable from a lack of oxygen, so, too, are your organs affected if you are oxygen-starved. They become sluggish. The organs of elimination—the lungs, kidneys, bowels, and skin—clog with waste. When they are overloaded, the accumulated wastes must go somewhere. For example, toxins pouring into your sweat glands begin to produce foul odors. The pores of the skin become clogged and unhealthy. Wastes are deposited in the mucous lining of your lungs, sinus cavities, throat, or nose.

When this happens you may say you "caught a cold" or "have the flu." Toxins can even be deposited into your joints and muscles, and you will begin to complain of spasms, soreness, or the pain of arthritis.

Perform a simple experiment. Place two lighted candles side by side. Cover one partially with a glass and observe the flame. What happens? It shrinks. What happens when you cover it completely? It goes out in a matter of seconds. Now think about what happens to your physical body when you deprive it of air. You can live about six minutes without air.

A Brighter Flame Is Possible

To achieve a brighter flame of life, you need more oxygen. Most of us take air for granted, and we have become shallow breathers. How would you react if, every time you sat down to a meal, someone pulled away three-quarters of it? Eventually, you would get mad and fight back before you starved to death! Yet most of us do exactly this every day with our most important nutrient, our air!

Makes you want to take a deep breath right now, doesn't it? So why not do yourself a favor? Stand up, feet shoulder-width apart, squarely planted. Bend your knees and bend forward from the waist. Just let your upper body hang for a few moments as you exhale. (You can feel the added benefit of taking the kinks out of your back.) Now, slowly rise and inhale a deep, satisfying breath as you reach up and try to touch the stars. Rise up on your toes. Exhale slowly. Repeat three times. This exercise is a good pick-me-up anytime during the day. It works better than caffeine pills or candy bars to revitalize your body and brain with oxygen.

Now that you're back, your brain is a little clearer, the most vital questions we can ask are "How do you increase your life force?" and "How is it related to oxygen?"

To raise your vibratory rate, you have to feed the trillions of cells that comprise your body with oxygen. One way to do this is through all the fresh fruits and vegetables you eat, particularly the leafy green vegetables and any green food supplements you may be taking, such as freshwater algaes like chlorella and spirulina, wheat grass, barley green, alfalfa, or blue-green algae. Fresh green foods and powdered green food supplements are rich with chlorophyll, which carries an abundance of oxygen into your body and feeds and detoxifies your cells. Another way is through deep breathing.

However, to increase your oxygen supply, eating plenty of green foods and deep breathing are good, but they are not enough. You must actively get the oxygen to those cells and there is only one sure way to do it.

You Have to Exercise!

Isn't it true that athletes seem to radiate more energy, more life force? It is because they exercise. If they also learn the lesson of dietary cleanliness and enzyme replacement, they have the potential to glow even more—and to extend their lives. Unfortunately, few of us are athletes. The truth is, we have become a nation of sitters and shallow breathers. Recent research indicates that nearly 80 percent of Americans are sedentary.

I believe that when anthropologists of the future examine the remains of the bodies of our century, they will name us *Homo sedentarius*. They'll most likely find a fossilized man with a remote control in one hand and a can of beer in the other. Life is motion. Hippocrates said, "To rest is to rust, and to rust is to decay."

But what is the best exercise? Is it walking? Of course, walking is excellent, and if you are not walking at least twenty minutes a day—as a deliberate form of rapid exercise or at a good clip to and from work—you are not taking advantage of one of your best opportunities to keep your legs, hips, and heart in shape. We repeat, you should make sure you walk briskly every day for at least twenty minutes. Your body was designed to do so. Our legs contain some of the largest muscles in our bodies, and they crave exercise. Boxers know that if they lose their legs, they lose the fight.

It is absolutely possible to walk and not necessarily raise your life force to its highest potential. Certain regions of the body *must* be exercised to raise your vitality, and walking actually weakens these muscles unless you take specific actions. The stomach is an example of a muscle that is weakened by walking. The stomach muscles, when you walk, actually tend to relax, while the lower back tightens and does the work. This is why many people will experience a sore back after excessive walking.

While reading this book, open and close your left hand rapidly for about a minute. What do you notice? It turns red with the glow of health. Feel the tingling? It is as if the millions of cells in your hand are saying "Thank You." However, you can't get this feeling of vitality in your hands just from walking. Walking does *nothing* to develop the muscles in the biceps and back, or the muscles of the triceps, shoulders, and chest. Walking burns fat, but it doesn't put the spine through its range of motion. Walking is great for the heart, but the heart is only one of about 640 muscles.

Beyond Walking: The Importance of Being Muscular

Exercise provides the heart with a fantastic support system. Every muscle is an "assistant" heart, helping to pump blood. When a muscle contracts, it squeezes blood toward the heart. When it relaxes, it allows the muscle to be filled with blood, exactly like the heart. Strong, healthy muscles take the burden off your heart. Think: Weak muscles, weak heart; strong muscles, strong heart.

Muscles grow strong and stay youthful with exercise. Sedentary behavior will cause your muscles to atrophy. This is a disease known as *sarcopenia*, or the loss of muscle tissue. As we age, the primary tissue we lose is muscle mass. The muscle mass of a thirty-year-old is less than that of a twenty-year-old, so the loss begins early.[5]

Many of the elderly in our country can't navigate a flight of stairs because their leg muscles aren't strong enough to carry them. Torturously, they lug their bodies around like dead weight because they have no muscle left to do the job. There is no need for muscle tone to *ever* be lost, but in our country we look at aging as a time of physical degeneration.

The Centers for Disease Control (CDC) predicts that over 50 percent of all Americans living today will spend their last years dying slowly in nursing homes, unable to care for themselves.[6] Fifty percent! One out of two! We believe much of this grim statistic can be attributed to cultural ignorance about the critical

---

[5]*Nutrition Action Healthletter.* Center for the Public Interest, December 1995, p. 4.
[6]Michael Colgan. "Four Nutrients to Stop Aging." *Muscular Development*, July 1994, p. 20.

need to *never* stop working the muscles of the body. We've become soft and sedentary television watchers and are paying the price. It doesn't have to be this way. Muscles will respond at any age; where there is the spark of life, there is hope.

In Asia and India, and even in much of Europe, the elderly are vital and active, and many are as muscular and toned as the young. Here, we specialize in the untoned muscle. It's flabby and lazy and rebels at performing. It wants only to "take it easy." A flabby muscle is an "old" muscle. If you want to restore youth and vitality, it's time to get your muscles working!

Lose Your Fear

Many people are afraid to exercise because they fear pain. What they don't understand is that they are in pain because of the lack of exercise.

Some even think that pain is normal, something they have to live with, and that it is a part of life. What most people experience as aches and pains, and believe is due to the natural course of aging, is Nature's way of telling us we are rusty and it is time to get off our backsides and work our muscles. By exercising our muscles we free them of tension and strengthen them. Often our pains are actually being caused by weak muscles that can't carry their share of the load.

Chiropractors and massage therapists, who work on the body in a hands-on way, know that one weak muscle—for example, one in the lower legs—can affect the knees and cause pain that will radiate upward. The body, trying to avoid the pain, throws itself off balance, which can then displace the hip and throw the spine out of alignment, ultimately causing headaches.

Again we can learn from our mentor, Jack LaLanne, who says, "As we age, many people complain about their muscles becoming stiff. It's the ligaments and tendons that connect the muscles to the bones. They are like rubber bands. If they are not used, they become brittle and lose their flexibility."[7]

LaLanne tells us that one of the best ways to overcome stiffness and aging is to do what children do almost unconsciously. Lie down on the floor. Stretch out. And then, immediately, get up! Does that feel awkward and stiff? Well, then keep doing it. Do it two times the first day, and work up slowly to ten or fifteen times.

This simple practice works every muscle in the body, and you'll find, much to your delight, that it becomes easier every day with practice. In other words, it restores you to a youthful body. As a result, every movement you make becomes easier. Do this exercise for a week, and then watch how much more fluid you are as you bend to pick up something you have dropped. In fact, tell yourself you can do one right now—and then do it! Make a game out of it. Do it with your children, your grandchildren, or your spouse.

"Use It or Lose It; to Rest Is to Rust"

We always tell our seminar groups: Your muscles will have plenty of time to rest in a coffin. Get up and LIVE!

Even the young are at risk of premature aging. It is not uncommon today to see children who have spent a sedentary day at school sitting in their homes after school and on the weekends, playing video games on computers or watching television. Less than two decades ago, these same children would have been outdoors riding bikes or playing basketball, baseball, or tennis. Schools across the nation are cutting physical education classes to save costs. Don't we realize that by denying our

---

[7]LaLanne. *Revitalize Your Life After Fifty*, p. 104.

children physical activity we are destroying their health? We see children who have stooped spines from lack of use.

Studying the most ancient forms of body dynamics, such as hatha yoga and Tai Chi Chuan, we discover they look to certain regions of the body as the most essential to exercise if you are going to increase your life force energies. Among the most crucial areas are the spine and the abdomen. The more recent martial arts, such as judo, aikido, karate, and tai kwan do, teach a similar philosophy of exercise.

Unfortunately, these disciplines are often designed for younger people of different cultures. The average sedentary American may find a lotus posture, or full Chinese splits, much too demanding! It is a truth, however, that we are as young or as old as our spines. It is also true that we judge our physical condition by the shape of our midsections.

You've learned the dangers of constipation in another chapter. The Japanese believe that our health, vitality, and sexual power can be determined by the strength of our abdomen. Our country suffers from an epidemic of prolapsed abdomens.

This means our intestines are sitting in our laps instead of being properly positioned. When the muscles are properly exercised and toned, waste material is properly moved along the intestines and out of the body. Restoring the abdomen to its position of power requires the use of exercise and a slant board.[8] Lying on a slant board, feet elevated above head, for at least ten minutes a day will help restore those organs to their natural place. It is also going to take two simple daily directed exercises to tone the stomach muscles.

---

[8]See the resource guide on page 373.

▼

DR. SCHNELL'S R. & D.

America has a national heritage of robust activity. Let's begin to recapture it. Before the jogging and aerobics era, and before health club memberships took exercise out of the home lifestyle, many of our Natural Health pioneers—Jack LaLanne, Charles Atlas, Paul Bragg, and Dr. Randolph Stone—used daily natural movements to keep their life force dynamic and their muscles young and active.

They have left us this legacy. Years ago, after working with these movements since my teens and studying the musculoskeletal system in chiropractic school, I compiled them into a naturally flowing series called BODYTONICS. You can use these exercises every day to increase your life force by stimulating and toning your whole body, particularly those regions that will bring you the most vitality.

If you have been feeling as if you needed something new in your exercise program, please see BODYTONICS as a basic foundation from which you can start every morning. If you have been absent from the exercise arena and are ready to begin, consult with your health care provider first. But please also refuse to listen to well-meaning "friends" or spouses who encourage you to remain sedentary. You don't need any encouragement to remain a "softy."

BODYTONICS can be done at any age or level of proficiency, because they are designed to allow you to work at your own pace, and within your personal range of motion. They can be done at any age or level of proficiency, because they are designed to allow you to work at your own pace, and within your personal range of motion. They can be done slowly and gently or at as demanding a speed and intensity as your body can handle. In this sense they are unique, designed to accommodate not only active Americans who are ready for quick and efficient, truly relevant exercise in their own homes, but also for those who wish to stop suffering the ravages of a sedentary existence. BODYTONICS are for everyone. Remember: the added benefit they bring is the raising of your life force, or spiritual vibrations, by pumping oxygen to every cell of your body.

A staggering quarter of a million deaths each year can be attributed solely to inactivity.[9] A sedentary lifestyle is as much a risk factor for disease as high blood pressure, obesity, and smoking.[10] Do you realize that watching a lot of

---

[9]Colgan. "American College of Sports Medicines." *Muscular Development*, July 27, 1993.
 [10]Ibid.

TV puts you in the same risk category as smokers? To rest is to rust, and to be sedentary is to be stagnant. To grow spiritually we must overcome this stagnation.

What can you do right now to make a new beginning? Sitting or standing, pretend you have a tight belt around your middle and attempt to pull your stomach in away from it. Hold your stomach muscle tightly pulled in for about five seconds. Then relax. Do this often, every time you think about it.

▲

**The Ninth Principle
of Natural Health and Weight Loss**

Cleanse and feed all the muscles of your body
every day by spending twelve to twenty minutes
in an active spine-based exercise routine.

Exercise As Sacred Personal Time

In many gyms we've turned the exercise arena into a "scene," or a place where the music would make you think you had entered a disco. In reality, exercise time is personal, a sacred time and space to forget about the world and its problems. It is the ideal time to clear the mind and concentrate solely on the muscle you are working. Through intense mental focus on the muscle being worked, both mind and body are strengthened. In fact, when we are exercising, we are working with the most sacred aspect of human existence, our life force.

The radiant energy of the life force creates an auric field around the body. Within this aura are lines of force, or energy pathways, along which your life force travels. They are related to the acupuncture meridians of Chinese medicine and to the nadis, the subtle nerve channels of the tantric/energy system of yoga. If one of our energy pathways becomes stagnant, we experience blocks or difficulties in a corresponding area of our body.

The old-time palm readers, and the modern philosopher George Gurdjieff, believed that these energy pathways were recorded on the palms. Modern-day practitioners of foot reflexology and iridology have a similar philosophy, and believe these energy pathways can be stimulated in the feet and observed in the eyes. These pathways may show on the hands and feet, but they emerge from our core—deep inside. When an energy pathway becomes blocked, a disease manifests. The same happens to water in a stream. If you obstruct the flow, you will get stagnant water.

Since the energy pathways emerge from the center of our being, if we want to keep them unobstructed, it makes sense to have an exercise program that is spine-based, which is one of the cornerstones of the BODYTONICS routine. The spine, after all, is the central structure of the human body. When you move the spine through its range of motion, you help prevent the mechanical blocks that may interfere with the flow of your life force.

▼

Using BODYTONICS, all your muscles and nerves are bathed in oxygen. Remember, your blood must carry nourishment and oxygen to your cells. With BODYTONICS, not only is your oxygenated blood feeding the cells, it is also cleansing them, picking up toxic by-products of cell metabolism, which Dr. John Tilden, author of *Toxemia Explained*, states is the root cause of all illness. A sluggish, sedentary body, made up of cells that never get fed and never get cleaned, is a body that will be sick.

▲

BODYTONICS removes the stagnation by exercising every muscle group from head to toe. If you're a beginner, you may start with only a few repetitions and be finished in five or ten minutes. As you become stronger, you'll find continued improvement from this routine by spending as little as twelve to twenty minutes a day. And if you are like us, you'll use your BODYTONICS routine, in part or in whole, *more* than once a day—as often, in fact, as you feel your energy lagging or your body becoming too sedentary.

Take your daily BODYTONICS seriously, as if your life depends on it, because it does! For the next thirty days, without fail, set aside ten to twelve minutes first thing in the morning to form your BODYTONICS habit. In thirty days, you'll find you're *addicted* to exercise. You'll find an indispensable feature of your day, as basic as the brushing of your teeth or eating, will be . . .

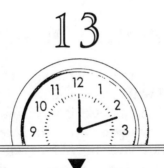

13

The 12‑Minute Daily BODYTONICS Routine

▼

► Before beginning any exercise program, check with your health care provider.

"Exercise stimulates the production of enzymes that convert fat to energy."
—Clarence Bass, *Lean for Life*

► Avoid exercise after eating. The best time for this quick routine is as a jumpstart in the morning, immediately after awakening. In this manner you set a tone of activity for the whole day.

► As you begin the BODYTONICS routine, you will notice that we are not recommending large numbers of repetitions to start. Most people fail in exercise programs because they try to do too much and then burn out and quit. With BODYTONICS, begin with a maximum of ten repetitions per movement. (Ten is the ideal. If you can do only three, then be satisfied with three and know that you will soon be doing more.) Be consistent every day and increase by a few repetitions every week.

BODYTONICS

▶ BODYTONICS are a very personal form of exercise. Unlike aerobics classes, where you must keep up with the group's tempo, with BODYTONICS it is absolutely imperative that you go at your own pace. At West Point and East Carolina University, studies have shown that self-paced exercise is superior to an artificial cadence established when someone else does the counting.[1] If your body is lazy in the beginning, you'll be able to coax it with fewer repetitions. On the other hand, on energetic days, you'll do more.

▶ BODYTONICS are composed of whole body movements. Whole body movements, as opposed to isolated body movements such as you see in other aerobics exercises, are another cornerstone of this routine. Whole body movements burn more calories than isolated movements, and they are better for your circulation. This means they are better for your heart.

▶ When performing BODYTONICS, use controlled movements and put your mind into your muscles. Focus on the muscles you are working. Many top athletes call this focus the "kinesthetic sense" and say it adds extra shape and tone to the muscle being worked. Dr. Kenneth Ravizza, a sports psychologist at California State University, maintains that awareness is the first step in raising self-control in any physical endeavor, and thus developing this awareness is a critical element of peak performance. This mind-muscle connection is a relatively new component in Western exercise programs. I've noticed all too frequently in health clubs throughout America that members are performing mindless exercise by flinging limbs or weights hither and thither in a totally unconscious manner, bringing little benefit and carrying a high risk of injury. In the long-lived Eastern cultures, the ap-

---

[1] P. F. Lachance and T. Hortogayi. *Strength and Conditioning Research,* vol. 8, no. 2, 1994.

proach toward exercise involves the totality of the individual. America is finally ready to tap into the mind-body-spirit connection in exercise.

▶ Many exercise programs assume that you have nothing but time on your hands. They require at least a ten-to-fifteen-minute warm-up; but with BODYTONICS, by the time ten or fifteen minutes have passed, you will have completed the entire daily routine. Keep in mind that if you can't make time for just twelve minutes, you are making time for illness.

▶ Most warm-ups involve some strenuous movements or a lengthy stretching routine. In this routine, the general warm-up of the muscle will take place during the exercise movement itself. Prior to that, what needs to be warmed or loosened are the joints that will be forced to bear the stress of the exercise.

The Joint Warm-up

NECK JOINT

We start with the neck joint and work down the body. This warm-up unlocks the facet joints of the neck. Flex the head forward, chin toward the chest, and then extend it gently backward and repeat for three to five repetitions. Be sure to arch the

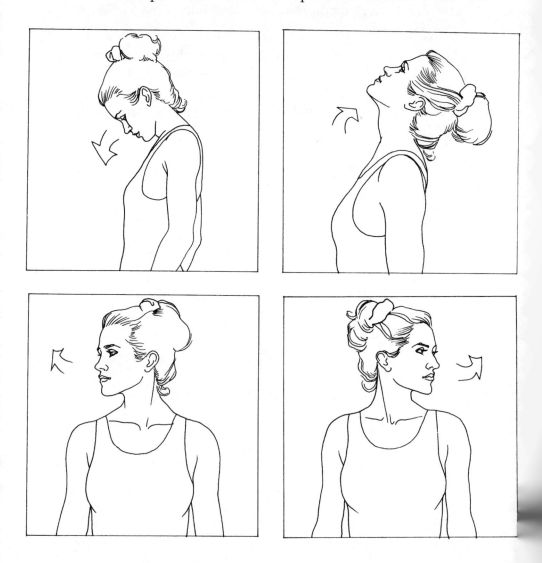

neck slightly upward when you move your head backward, so as not to pinch or overly shorten the back of your neck. Now turn the head and look over the right shoulder three to five times, and then the left shoulder.

In doing this, imagine that your neck and head are on a long pole and that your neck rotates directly on the pole. Avoid a side-to-side tilting of your head.

SHOULDER JOINTS

Place your hands on your shoulders, elbows out to the sides, and rotate the arms in a forward direction, forming large circles with the elbows. Do three to five repetitions, and then reverse, taking the shoulders and elbows backward in large circles.

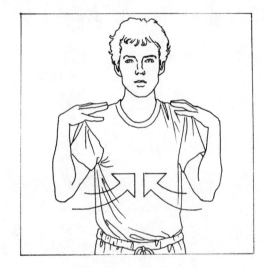

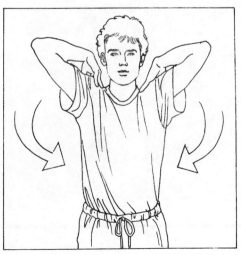

ELBOW JOINTS

We unlock the elbow joints by stabilizing the left elbow with the right hand behind and slightly above the joint. Rotate forearm three to five times, making circles toward the body with the palm facing down. Rotate the elbow joint only in this direction. Do both arms.

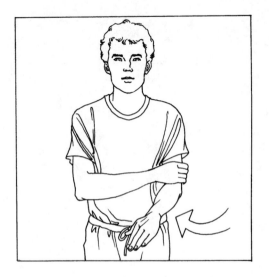

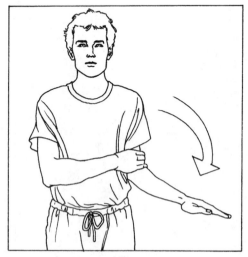

WRIST JOINTS

Stabilize the wrist joints in the same way, rotating them three to five times clockwise and counterclockwise.

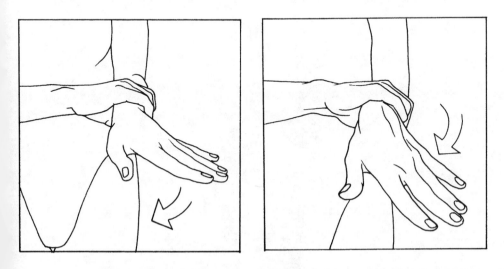

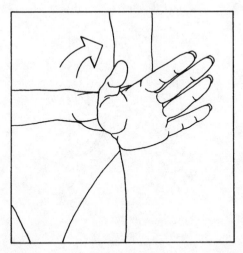

SPINAL JOINTS

Place your hands on your hips with your knees slightly bent.
Rotate your upper body, above the hips, three to five times
clockwise and counterclockwise. This provides a gentle freeing
of the lumbar spine and starts to free the sacrum.

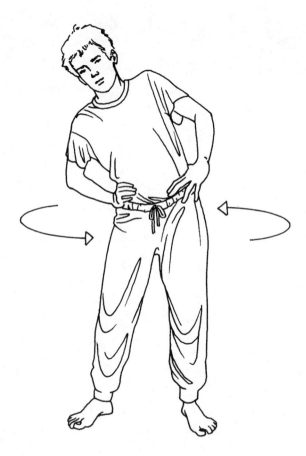

HIP JOINTS

Stand with feet firmly planted, eighteen inches apart, knees slightly bent, hands on hips. Keep your upper body stationary and rotate your hips, Elvis-style, three to five times in each direction. This gives more freedom of movement to the lumbar/sacral region.

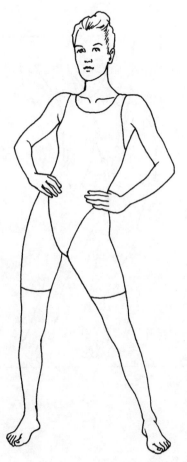

KNEES AND ANKLE JOINTS

Place your hands above your knees, knees slightly bent, feet a few inches apart, and rotate the knees clockwise and counterclockwise, three to five times in each direction. Knees and legs are rotating. Hands are stabilizing.

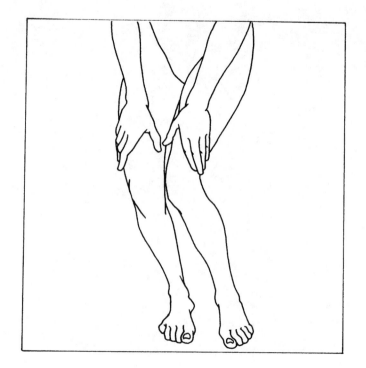

BODYTONICS Routine

THE NECK SHAPER

WHY:

The neck is your appearance muscle. It's the one part of the body everyone can see, so it pays to keep it toned. The skull is so much heavier than we realize. It can weigh between five and seven pounds. Many people suffer headaches because their neck muscles are too weak and flabby to hold their heads properly. The lack of muscular development predisposes them to poor posture and neck injuries. You will be working all of the muscle groups of the body from the neck down, and by starting with the neck you are signaling your medulla, your internal control switch at the base of your brain, that physical activity is being demanded from you.

One of the most common ailments that affects the elderly is senility, the deterioration of mental faculties. It has often been observed by bodyworkers and physical therapists that there is a direct correlation between the musculoskeletal health of a person's neck and that person's level of mental functioning. It doesn't surprise us that we are a nation in need of an abundance of headache remedies. Perhaps regular exercise of the neck region will, over time, keep the brain healthier and you more alert.

HOW:

Place your palms against your forehead with fingers extending off the top of your head, creating light "fingertip resistance." Bring the chin to the chest and then up to a neutral position, eyes straight ahead, breathing out while exerting. Do only five repetitions. The neck is a small muscle and tires easily, and this is one area you don't want to overwork. Now place your hands behind your head, again with light resistance. Take the chin

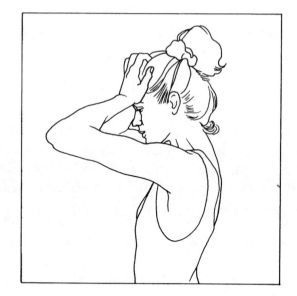

from the chest backward to a neutral position with the eyes looking straight ahead. Do five repetitions.

BEAR SWING

WHY:
The Bear Swing gives the spin a gentle side-to-side rotation to begin to warm up the back and stomach. Its movements take the rust out of your spine. The Bear Swing helps to reduce tension in the shoulder muscles, which connect into the neck. Almost everyone carries a high level of shoulder tension. This is where you often carry your burdens, "shoulder" responsibilities, and "support the weight of the world." The Bear Swing tones the sides of the waist, the love handles—what we like to call the "croissant muscle."

HOW:
With arms loosely outstretched and legs shoulder-width apart, begin twisting with the torso, looking behind you at the end of

each repetition. Breathe as you move. Put your breath into the motion. No more oxygen starvation for you! Start with ten and work up to twenty or more over a month's time.

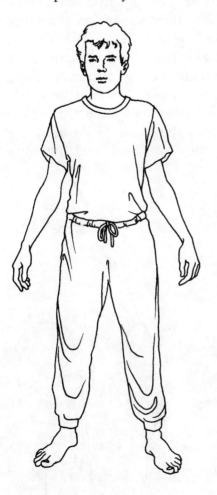
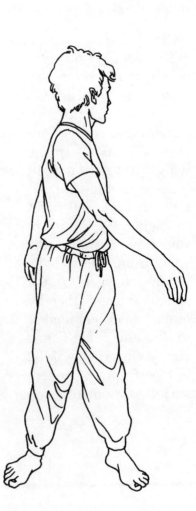

CHURNING

WHY:

With the Bear Swing, you gave your spine a gentle side-to-side warm-up. Now you are ready for churning, which is a more active working of the same muscle group. You're going to recruit more muscle fibers to get the job done, which means better toning benefits. This is a familiar movement; you most likely did it in physical education classes when you were in grade school. People don't realize what tremendous relief it brings to a tired back. This movement tones the backs of the legs, the sides of the waist, the stomach, the lower back, and the inner thigh.

HOW:

With feet shoulder-width apart, bend forward at the waist at a 90-degree angle, hold your stomach in, arms outstretched, like airplane wings. Touch your right hand to your left toe and then alternate left hand to right toe. You are smoothly turning the spine from side to side, sending oxygen to the spinal nerves, thereby toning them. Remember to breathe. Don't just flail your arms wildly, but perform controlled, smooth movements.

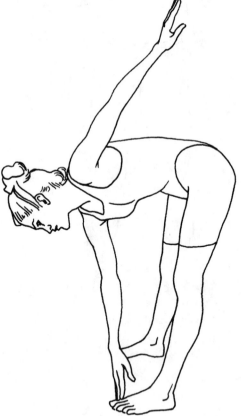

BRAGGING

WHY:

When we were developing the BODYTONICS routine, we paid particular attention to what the health and fitness pioneers did for their own exercise. We were mostly interested in the fitness routines of those who lived actively into their nineties or beyond. This movement as well as the others kept coming up as a favorite.

Too often, as people start to age, they get a stooped, stiff look because they have lost the forward-backward mobility of the spine. It is the appearance of a degenerating condition taking over from lack of use, and Bragging can prevent it. This was a favorite exercise of Dr. Paul Bragg, who lived a long, active life—surfing in his nineties!

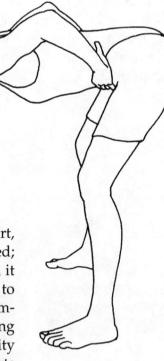

HOW:

Place your feet shoulder-width apart, hands on hips, knees slightly flexed; bend the upper body forward until it is parallel to the floor, then return to an upright position. This is a warm-up motion to start gradually restoring the forward and backward mobility of your spine. Bragging also starts to unlock the sacrum. Do ten and breathe.

WOODCHOPPER

WHY:

Having warmed up our spines with Bragging, we are now able to move into a more vigorous motion. This exercise works all the muscle groups of the body and is particularly effective for the lower back and sacrum.

The Woodchopper has important spiritual implications as well. As we have said, the spiritual and healing practices of the Eastern cultures believe the life force is located at the base of the spine, in the sacrum. This exercise is wonderful for bringing an abundant supply of oxygen to this region. The Woodchopper tones the stomach muscles as well.

HOW:

Start with your feet slightly wider than shoulder width, with the knees bent. Clasp your hands in front of you, bring them up as if you're raising an ax, and then bring them down between your legs as if you are chopping wood. The Woodchopper is performed in a smooth, controlled fashion, allowing the spine to lengthen.

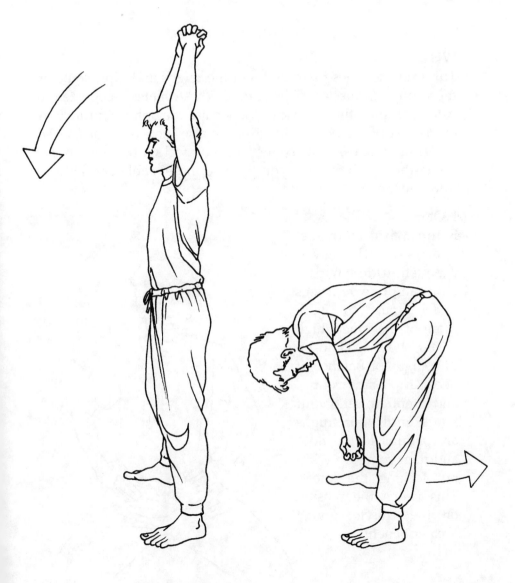

THIGH SHAPER

WHY:

This exercise tones the muscles of the thighs and hips, some of the strongest muscles in the entire body. Athletes recognize the value of toning these muscles to increase the optimum function of the rest of the body. This exercise also increases your sense of "groundedness," the connection you feel with the earth. By doing the Thigh Shaper, you become more stable and able to fully function in the world.

HOW:

Stand with your feet apart, slightly wider than shoulder width. (You can place your legs wider apart to work more of the inner thigh if you choose.) Hold on to a chair for balance, if necessary. Using control and intention, bend your knees until your thighs are parallel to the floor and then come up without locking the knees. This keeps the tension on the muscle, giving greater benefit.

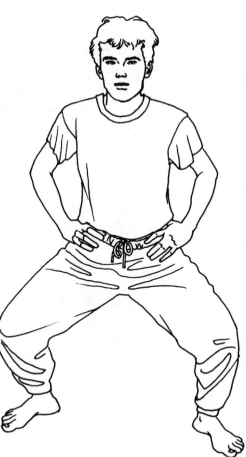

BUN SHAPER

WHY:

Karate instructors have long taught the importance of toned buttocks muscles for punching power. Watch professional baseball players and you will notice that they get their batting power from the powerful rotation of the trunk, which is the job of the buttocks. This exercise brings a surplus of oxygen to the sacral plexus. The nerves in this region get bathed with oxygen-rich blood. This is of vital importance because these nerves control our sexual health as well as the nerves to the lower colon, for elimination.

HOW:

The Bun Shaper can be done on the floor or on a stool. Lie on your stomach across a stool and grasp the legs of the stool. Lift your legs, pause, and contract the buttocks. This exercise should be done one leg at a time until you're strong enough to lift both legs at the same time. The Bun Shaper strengthens and tones the muscles of the buttocks, hamstrings, and lower back.

This exercise is a favorite of Jack LaLanne, who is still going strong.

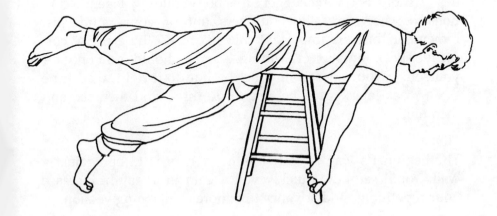

CHEST SHAPER

WHY:

As people age, one of the problems associated with the sedentary lifestyle is the loss of strength in the upper body. This is really a loss of muscle tissue that scientists call *sarcopenia*. The Chest Shaper quickly rebuilds upper body strength by working the back, shoulders, arms, chest, and wrists.

Women don't normally think they are able to pull their upper body weight, but that capability is not related to gender. Rather, it's the result of the lack of training, or nonuse. The Chest Shaper is a modified push-up. It tones the back, shoulders, backs of the arms, and chest muscles. It's not going to build a bulky appearance because it is a *natural movement.*

When we say "natural," we are referring to the idea that, to survive in Nature, you have to be able to pull your own weight. That's why the Chest Shaper is so important. It gradually restores the upper body strength that most women (and men) in our culture have lost.

Jack LaLanne once performed over a thousand repetitions of this exercise in only twenty minutes. This exercise was also a favorite of Charles Atlas, who was doing 250 a day in his nineties. Arnold Schwarzenegger, the bodybuilding legend, cautions us, however: "Put numbers out of your mind. Just remember this: the important thing is to do the exercise correctly. That counts for everything. . . . You should train only for yourself. If you can do only one . . . but do it right, that's fine . . . a week later, you'll be able to do three, and then six, and then ten."[2]

HOW:

The beginner's way to start this movement is to be against a wall. You'll see how quickly you'll gain in strength, increase your repetitions, and advance to a more challenging version.

---

[2]Arnold Schwarzenegger. *Arnold: The Education of a Bodybuilder.* New York: Simon & Schuster, 1977, pp. 162–63.

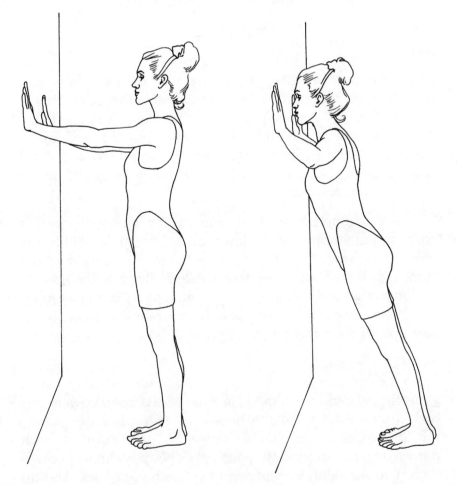

Stand at arm's length from the wall and place your hands on the wall directly in front of you at shoulder level. Place your feet a comfortable distance apart. Inhale and, bending your elbows outward, attempt to touch your chest to the wall. Put your mind into the muscle and feel it work.

Now exhale and push off in a controlled, smooth movement without locking the elbows. Keep your hips in line with your upper body. Most people will need to start with between five and ten of these movements. When you have built up to two sets of ten, try a few repetitions on the floor, perhaps on your knees before you attempt the full-length traditional version.

FIT-UPS

WHY:

Americans need a fast and effective way to strengthen their stomachs—or, more properly, their abdominal muscles. Part of the epidemic of low back problems in this country is due to the state of our overly soft and flabby midsections. The abdominal muscles act as a support system for the low back, and if the abdominal muscles are weak, too much strain is placed on the muscles of the low back.

It is also important to strengthen the abdomen in a way that does not put strain onto the lower back. There is a muscle, the psoas, that travels from the inside of the thigh, across the front of the pelvis area, and then deep inside to attach to the front of the lumbar spine. If done incorrectly, abdominal exercises strain this muscle, thereby causing low back strain and possibly injury. Follow the directions carefully on this one.

HOW:

Sit on the floor, on the edge of a pillow you have placed beneath you. Slightly bend your knees, feet flat on the floor. Lower your body backward toward the floor until it touches the pillow, inhaling, focusing on your abdomen. Then perform a crunch motion as you curl up until your upper body is almost perpendicular to the floor. Remember: Don't arch your back, and do exhale as you go down.

You might have heard that the only abdominal exercise to perform is the "crunch." Crunches are an isolated movement, and most beginners don't have the strength to perform them properly. We've done thousands of crunches, but we love Fit-ups because they give us the benefits of the crunch and a traditional sit-up combined into one movement.

Fit-ups also give us a coiled, tight feeling in our midsections. You feel your personal power increase almost after the first few repetitions. Before the discovery of the crunch and its push at health clubs, Charles Atlas, Arnold Schwarzenegger, and Jack LaLanne all had impeccable midsections from using sit-ups.

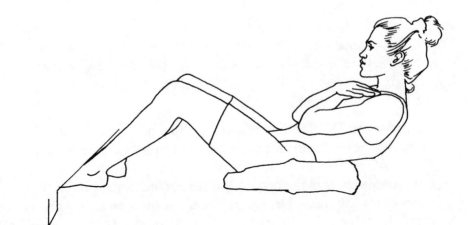

You may have never heard of Irwin Koszewski. He's won more awards for best abdominals than anyone in history. In his seventies, he still does a thousand full sit-ups every day. According to Steve Holman, author of *Critical Mass*, contrary to popular belief, the sit-up targets most of the abdominal muscles.

The one complaint many crunch experts have about sit-ups is that they involve the hip flexor muscles in the legs to a great degree. In Holman's opinion, that's an asset, not a liability. He says the muscle teamwork allows you to recruit the most muscle fibers and concludes: "If you want the fastest abdominal development, you should include sit-ups as well as leg raises."[3] Which brings us to our next BODYTONIC.

---

[3]"Sit-ups Superiority." *Ironman Magazine,* August 1994, p. 41.

FIT-DOWNS

WHY:

This is a leg raise and completes the strengthening of the abdominal muscles and the lower back. It is another exercise that builds spiritual power. The martial arts focus intensely on strengthening this region.

According to Dr. Ramurti Mishra, author of *Fundamentals of Yoga*, the abdomen is an important seat of spiritual power because it contains the solar plexus. Mishra, a psychiatrist, taught that the solar plexus is the center of our subconscious mind and is a battery for life force. Dr. Hugh Greer Carruthers, a psychiatrist and founder of the Theological Science Society, believed this as well. These enlightened physicians believed that we store our surplus life force in this region.

So, if you are feeling low in vitality, do some Fit-ups and Fit-downs to bring the blood that carries the life force to your solar plexus battery.

HOW:

Lit flat on the floor, on your back, hands along your sides or palms down under your hips, feet together. Bend your knees together, bring them up to your chest, and push them straight out. Breathe throughout the movement.

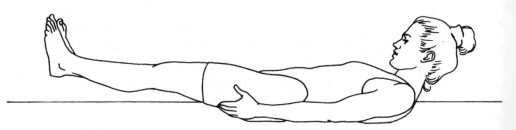

BICEP BUILDER

WHY:
Now you return to a standing position; you will be doing a couple of isolated movements to cool down and gently stimulate the blood to return to the heart. Although we think of the heart as the muscle that pumps blood, don't forget that the arms and legs are also pump muscles, and they can take the burden off the heart. This exercise also brings tone and shape to the upper arms.

HOW:
Grasp your left wrist with your right hand. Starting with your arm at a 120° angle, curl your left arm toward your shoulder, applying gentle resistance with your right hand. Contract your upper arm at the top, and control the movement going down. Put your mind into your muscle.

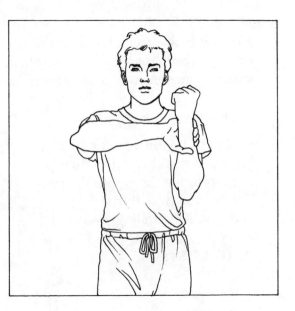

CALF SHAPER

WHY:

This is the final movement to tone the muscles of the lower legs and to strengthen the ankles and pump the blood back to the heart. The Calf Shaper is a wonderful exercise for women who wear high heels—heels tend to shorten the muscle, and the Calf Shaper will tend to correct this. It is also great for joggers, tennis players, skiers, and all athletes, because if the calf muscle, Nature's shock absorber, is developed, it can handle more force and protect the knees.

HOW:

Hold on to the back of a chair and rise up on your toes in a controlled, smooth movement, contracting the calf muscles at the top. Slowly return your heels to the ground.

That's it. You've done it! Now feel your body and the life force pulsing through it. Stay with the routine for the next thirty days and you'll be telling everyone you know: **TO REST IS TO RUST!**

PART FOUR

THE FITONICS™ FORMULA FOR HIGH-ENERGY EATING

14

▼

It's Time for Action

▼

*"Sometimes I feel like I've eaten more than I should have
or eaten something I shouldn't have eaten,
and I'll think, 'Oh, I'm going to get on the scale,
and I'll have gained weight,'
and every time I'll have lost another pound.
It's just amazing.
I feel like the weight's just falling off.
I've been at this weight for eleven years,
since I had my last child.
I've done all kinds of diets and have been successful,
but most diets have you change
the way you're eating while you're on the diet.
So, you don't eat this, you don't eat that,
and then you're always looking forward to when
the diet is going to be over and you can eat
other food again.
With FITONICS you're not doing that.
Marilyn's recipes are so wonderful,
you look forward to a meal,
and when on a diet do you look forward to a meal?"*

—KITTY W.
(interviewed at the end of the FITONICS test;
lost twenty-one pounds in eight weeks)

On the following pages, you will find a review of the FITONICS High-Energy Eating strategies and principles. Then you'll be ready to spring into action with the recipes you'll need to prepare the recommended meals. See this program as your step to empowerment over the foods you eat and the positive results they bring to your life. Once you have mastered your new approach to eating, you'll have this program at your fingertips for the rest of your life. With mastery of the principles, *food becomes your friend.*

Three days of sample menus have been specially designed to help you understand how to apply the FITONICS principles in your kitchen and how to make them a natural part of the way you eat. In adhering closely to the recommendations, you'll see the success you're seeking in the shortest possible time. Of special interest to those who have limited time for shopping or kitchen preparation, we have included the satisfying and slenderizing ONE-DISH MEALS, all of which are a breeze to put together, and which give us the energy to truly enjoy our lives.

For example:

▶ *The "TONIC" in all its variations—A breakfast in a glass for those on the run, wanting more time for fun.*

▶ *Fruit "Cereals"*—Slenderizing blends of fresh fruits, dried nuts, and milks that are live, live, live!

▶ *High-Energy Super-Salads*—The Philly Cheese Steak Salad, Thai Chicken Salad, and Farmer's Chop Suey—the most satisfying way we have found for adding more live food to our daily diet.

▶ *Soothing Suppers*—Comforting "bowls" of Mashed Potatoes and Gravy, Angel Hair Pasta with Chicken and Spinach or the satisfying Soup and Sweet Dinner, our special secret for making the sweets we love a healthful part of our lives.

Finally, we address one of the most common concerns on the health scene today as we review our personal formula for sensible supplementation.

As You Believe, You Receive

We've given you all the rationales we have gathered from our lifetime studies of Natural Health for the actions you will now be taking. As you eat menus based on pure, natural foods, and as you increase the live food in your diet, expect to lose weight and feel increasingly energetic. You may also experience a "detoxification" and rejuvenation of body and mind, so your spirit can begin to shine through more brightly than ever.

Detoxification may carry with it a few days of headaches as you move away from caffeine in coffee and sodas, or the tendency to urinate or move your bowels more frequently as your body begins to cleanse. All these symptoms will pass quickly. Remember, they are the signs of returning health!

Expect a FITONICS Makeover!

The results you want will come from alignment with Natural Health principles and from your own mental, as well as physical, efforts. Those with the highest expectations for success will reap the greatest rewards. This idea is so important to your long-term transformation that it bears repeating: To reach your goals, you must first cultivate an expectation for success.

And a willingness to participate in that success. Unless you're willing to put in some effort on your own behalf in the kitchen, it will be harder to achieve the results you are seeking. We cannot urge you strongly enough during this wonderful phase of your life, as you reclaim your highest level of health and vitality, to *value* the time you spend on food shopping and food preparation. One of the most beautiful aspects of the human experience is the aroma-filled kitchen. It brings us the promise of joyful good eating, family happiness, and contentment that all is well in the home.

No More Food Guilt

The FITONICS formula is an easily implemented program, designed to remove the guilt and confusion that surround so much of the American eating experience. Since many of the comfort foods we were raised on have now been put on the "bad" list, it is time, as responsible and free-thinking adults, to let go of the guilt and begin, with confidence, to take positive action.

There are many foods we now know to be health building. At the top of this list of wholesome foods, including grains, legumes, lean meats, poultry, fish, and pure dairy, are fresh fruits and vegetables. As long as we eat *more* fruits and vegetables than any of the others, we are building health. In other words, it is not necessary to exclude any of the macro-nutrients (fats, carbohydrates, and proteins), but it is important to realize that *for that clean, light, young feeling, fruits and vegetables are the keys.*

Pure dairy meals include real butter, whole yogurt, *real* cheeses, and the nontraditional dairy products our forefathers and mothers enjoyed. Small, *reasonable* amounts of these foods satisfy us and keep us from bingeing on empty snack foods.

Proteins should be eaten in smaller amounts earlier in the day so that the body has a chance to digest them. Eaten at night, they can be both stimulating, as they rev up your metabolism, and heavy to digest as your body moves toward sleep.

Complex carbohydrates are most healthful when they are unrefined. Since they cause the release of serotonin in the brain, they are the perfect evening meal choice.

Thus, we recommend the Power Lunch of proteins and salads and the Soothing Supper of complex carbohydrates and vegetables.

You're in the Driver's Seat

We urge you to take a personal stand on what you desire to include in your own health regimen. Only you know what you need based on your upbringing and environment. As you begin to develop your own personal health regimen, the best tip we can give you is: **Stay flexible.** It is our experience that no one dietary philosophy works all the time for any individual. There will be times when you will religiously honor the principles we have offered, time for vegetarianism, time for meat eating, time for your Funday when you cleanse with live food.

We cannot encourage you enough to take the opportunity to cleanse your body on live food—especially in warm weather—one day a week. This is one of the best ways to stay vibrant and healthy, and to keep your weight right where you want it.

No More "Food Cops"

We have frequently heard advocates of vegetarian, vegan (a diet without any animal-based foods), or live food lifestyles judge those around them and lament family and social gatherings because their dietary preferences were compromised. We ourselves experienced the alienation, loneliness, and limitation that come from holding diet above human relationships and emotional needs. We would never advocate that you become so obsessed with your eating preferences that you allow them to rule your social interactions or the quality of your family life.

And, we ask you not to judge others. No more "food cops." Live and let live. The best you can do for those you love is set the example for Natural Health by radiating love and happiness.

There Is a Time and a Place for Everything

We cannot stress enough that it is a perfectly normal aspect of human existence to celebrate and relate socially over food. Using rigid dietary philosophies as a justification to sacrifice those occasional opportunities for the natural customs of feasting, or "letting off steam," may take a toll on your psychological and emotional well-being that is not worth the physical benefit.

Our purpose is to help you avoid the mistake of becoming so rigid about your health goals that you forfeit some of the most important and rewarding aspects of human health: your family, social relationships, celebrations, and holidays.

And as an integral part of your journey toward health, give yourself the opportunity to relax and stretch out! Make your journey a pleasant experience all along the way. Enjoy the view! Stop and breathe deeply of the fresh, cool air. This is a lifetime endeavor. Not a jail sentence.

With FITONICS, we have done our best to give you simple guidelines to allow you to flow with your dietary options so your experience on the road to Natural Health is always enjoyable.

15

▼

A Review of the FITONICS Principles of Natural Health and Weight Loss

▼

1
ᔕᕇ

KEEP THE COLON CLEAN WITH FRESH FRUIT, VEGETABLES, AND HIGH-FIBER GRAINS OR LEGUMES.

You can do this by eating one live (raw) fruit or vegetable meal every day. This will keep your energy high and weight down. Choose from a variety of fresh fruit and vegetable juices, and the healthful tonics we recommend are excellent breakfast options. If you do decide to eat a heavier breakfast, have a fruit or salad meal at lunch or dinner. We have supplied ideas for wholesome alternatives to the fruit meal in the morning (see recipe section).

2

⟅∼⟆

TO KEEP ENZYME SUPPLIES HIGH AND ENERGY
ABUNDANT, AND TO SUPPORT WEIGHT LOSS, EAT *ONE* LIVE
FOOD MEAL EVERY DAY, CONSISTING SOLELY OF FRESH
FRUITS OR VEGETABLES.

This is extremely successful if you choose the tried-and-proven "fruit in the morning." Or you can opt for a fruit or salad meal at lunch or dinner. However, allow yourself the opportunity to experience the cleansing effect of fruit in the morning. Not only will you feel energized, but this will also bring about weight loss and end constipation.

3

⟅∼⟆

TO IMPROVE DIGESTION AND GET THE MOST FROM FOOD,
WE TAKE ENZYME SUPPLEMENTS WITH
EVERY COOKED MEAL.

Regular enzyme supplements can make a significant difference in general health, well-being, and, consequently, weight loss. This option offsets costly withdrawals from your enzyme bank account and helps expedite digestion. This is not a requirement of the program. It is simply one more tool from which you can benefit.

4

❧

TO LOSE WEIGHT AND INCREASE ENERGY, AVOID
ROUTINELY MIXING PROTEINS AND STARCHES. HAVE
PROTEINS WITH SALADS AND NONSTARCHY VEGETABLES
AT LUNCH (THE POWER LUNCH) AND STARCHES WITH
VEGETABLES AND/OR SALADS AT DINNER
(THE SOOTHING SUPPER).

Your POWER LUNCH allows you to eat stimulating protein foods with salads early in the day, when you need the mental stimulation and clarity protein foods provide. In the evening, your SOOTHING SUPPER mellows you out for relaxation, Hypno-Meditation, and a sound night's sleep.

Limit your animal protein—such as meat, chicken, eggs, or fish—to *once* a day if possible. For best results, eat animal flesh protein only three or four times a week. In other words, have some vegetarian days.

Please don't make the mistake of turning food combining into a law you must obey at all costs. We've heard the lament for pizza a thousand times over the past decade from those following the food combining principles in *FIT FOR LIFE* and religiously denying themselves all the foods they loved—until they ultimately rejected a tool they had turned into a rule. If you are craving pizza, have it. *We* do!

You should realize that there will be times you will mix proteins and starches, and times you won't. *It's entirely up to you.* With FITONICS, you can once and for all time let go of the idea that someone is looking over your shoulder every time you pick up a fork. No more "food cop" thinking!

5

༻

TO KEEP BODIES HEALTHFULLY ALKALINE, ENJOY A
FUNDAY AS OFTEN AS POSSIBLE, EATING ONLY FRESH,
UNCOOKED, NATURAL FOODS SUCH AS FRUITS,
VEGETABLES, SPROUTS, SUN-DRIED FRUITS, AND FRESH
JUICE.

In the winter, warm vegetable broths and cooked vegetables can help satisfy the need for warm food and go a long way to flushing the acids from the body. In the summer, take advantage of live food meals and Fundays. Other alkaline foods include soy milk, tofu, tempeh, lima and aduki (azuki) beans, almonds, and herbal teas to name just a few.

When we first stepped onto the road of Natural Health, we would take ten days at a time and eat only fresh fruit, vegetables, and juices. This is called monodieting. Once we felt our bodies were restored, we would then eat a regular daily balance of cooked and live food meals, interspersed with live food days. Today, whenever we find ourselves eating heavier foods, or whenever we feel our energy drop, we focus on live foods and simple vegetable meals. Above all, every year, we regularly make sure we take a few days to a week to a month for fruit-and-vegetable cleansing.

The Funday, when you drink only juices or tonics, or eat only fresh fruits and vegetables, is a valuable tool for a spring cleaning of your body. It is what you will rely on to offset any heavy eating you can't avoid or regroup after a celebration or vacation. It makes tremendous sense during the warm months, when your appetite for cooked foods is offset by the weather. When it is extremely hot, you might feel like a FUN *WEEK!*

Even though, on this program, we encourage you to take an occasional day on fruits and vegetables, we want you to know that the more days you take, the faster you'll reach your goal. You can have a day just on juice, a day when you eat only oranges and finished with a big mixed salad. You can start your day with fruit, have a salad at lunch, and then finish with more fruit or a bowl of cooked vegetables at supper. However you put your Funday together, make sure you are comfortable and satisfied with it.

6

THINK TWICE BEFORE USING SUGAR AND ARTIFICIAL INGREDIENTS.

There are many alternative whole food sweeteners now available in natural food stores. Sucanat, brown rice sugar, and date sugar are only a few. (See Resource Guide for mail-order sources.) These sweeteners provide nutrients as well as sweetness and can be used on cereals and in cooking and baking. Use honey to sweeten your tea.

Just as it is important to read labels for ingredients, it is imperative to read warning labels regarding highly artificial ingredients such as aspartame and olestra. Be aware of the symptoms these additives may cause.

7

TO ENSURE HEALTH AND HAPPINESS, MAKE A REGULAR EFFORT, ESPECIALLY FIRST THING IN THE MORNING, TO MENTALLY SET THE TONE FOR THE DAY.

If you do not "program" yourself for a positive outcome and tranquility you can be sure someone else will program you, and it may not be to your best advantage.

8

TO FIND PEACE AND HARMONY, TAKE 5 TO 20 MINUTES
EACH DAY TO DEEPLY RELAX BODY AND MIND.

Science has shown us that those who regularly use this principle reduce their risk of illness—mental and physical. The spiritual benefits cannot be measured.

CLEANSE AND FEED ALL THE MUSCLES OF YOUR BODY
EVERY DAY BY SPENDING 12 TO 20 MINUTES IN AN ACTIVE
SPINE-BASED EXERCISE ROUTINE.

This active routine in the morning can ready you for the demands of your day. Slower, more meditative spine-based exercise such as yoga or tai chi will mellow you out in the evening.

THE NINE FITONICS PRINCIPLES OF
NATURAL HEALTH AND WEIGHT LOSS
WILL GUIDE YOU ON ONE OF THE MOST IMPORTANT
AND PLEASURABLE JOURNEYS OF YOUR LIFE.

16

▼

How Much Should I Eat? Or Be Careful Not to Exceed the "Feed Limit"[1] and Other TIPS FOR SUCCESS

▼

Chew, Chew, Chew

Dr. Horace Fletcher wrote the first bestselling diet book in the late 1800s. He taught that the key to weight loss and health was to chew each mouthful one hundred times, until the food became a liquid. Common sense tells you that the more you chew your food, the less work your stomach has to do. There's a savings not only in energy but also in digestive enzymes. We're not asking you to chew your food a hundred times, but we are hoping you will break the habit of "bolting" down your food by reminding yourself as often as possible to "fletcherize" your food.

---

[1]A phrase from Natural Health pioneer Jack LaLanne.

Eat Regularly

If your natural pattern of eating is something you would like to improve upon, one of the best hints we can give you is: EAT REGULARLY. Avoid waiting until you are famished. Have a schedule. Know that you eat breakfast about this time, lunch about that time, and supper at that time. Make the meals small, especially if you are a woman. Women eat about half to two-thirds of what most men are capable of eating.

So you can give him a large bowl of soup, and you take a smaller one. Give him a whole sandwich (and a generous-sized one, at that), and give yourself half. Generally speaking, when it comes to salad and vegetables, women can easily eat twice the portion a man eats, but men will always want more meat and potatoes than women.

For women, use the "Palm Rule" as the "rule of thumb" to gauge protein portion sizes. The ideal serving of protein should not be greater than the size of your palm (fingers not included).

Most men will require more than that. Remember that men need protein and small amounts of fat to build testosterone. Women need protein for shiny hair and radiant skin and fat for the making of estrogen.

Between meals, have a small snack. For example, if you have a Tonic in the morning, have some fresh or dried fruit at mid-morning. If you have a salad and a piece of fish at lunch, wait three hours and then have more fruit. Or have a plain yogurt, one or two high-fiber crackers spread with avocado or almond butter, or fresh vegetable juice as a snack. In the evening, three hours after a dinner of starches and vegetables, and before bed, you may crave a banana, which will help you sleep.

The capacity of the average stomach is approximately a quart. Fill your stomach two-thirds to three-quarters full, and leave some space for the *prana*, or life energy, that allows the food to move around and digest. If you cram your stomach full, it's like overloading a washing machine or dryer. The food you have eaten will feel like it's stuck, and as all your energy goes toward digestion, you may feel irritable and grumpy.

Eat Light

If you are not hungry, have only as much as you crave. But *start with the salad*, or the vegetable, and then add heavier items. If you eat the heavier items and leave out the salad or vegetable, you lose the weight-loss benefit.

Keep It Simple

Keep your meals simple for better digestion. Those who eat simply have fewer problems with weight and disease and greater longevity. The famous Cornell-China-Oxford Study pioneered by Dr. T. Colin Campbell proved this point unequivocally. Chinese peasants, with their simple diets and active lives, are among the healthiest people in the world. For this reason, we advise: Serve a protein and a salad; a starch and vegetables.

Meal Options

The recipe section offers vegetarian and nonvegetarian meal options, giving you a chance to fully experience vegetarian eating if you desire. However, we urge you to make the choice *for health*, and not to make the mistake of embracing vegetarian eating to be part of an "in crowd" trend.

Vegetarianism for the wrong reasons can often be a risk to health. Those who are lacking a focus on health may tend to fill the void they have created in giving up animal proteins and dairy with white flour pasta, bread, and lots of sugary sweets.

This is, sadly, what many trend-following teenagers are now doing, and if you have a son or daughter who fits into this category, you will find balanced vegetarian recipes to answer their need for nutrients.[2]

The truth is, we can be perfectly healthy not being vegetarians. And, although being a vegetarian is an excellent choice, there is no guarantee that you will be healthy doing so—unless you pay strict attention to the quality of foods you are eating. First and foremost, eat for health!

Reverse Order

To suit your needs, lunch and dinner can be reversed and substituted one for the other. If you are cooking for your family, make enough protein at lunch to be able to serve those wishing to eat protein at the evening meal. For those not interested in food combining (i.e., children), the protein can complement the simple grain and vegetable meal you have prepared.

Substitutions

At any meal, feel free to substitute fruit, a salad, or a bowl of soup for the menu suggestions. These menus are to acquaint you with healthful recipes from a wide variety of ingredients. We suggest them because we believe a broad diet from many food sources guarantees you a better chance for good nutrition.

Repeat Foods

If you like one particular lunch or supper, feel free to repeat it.

---

[2]See also *The American Vegetarian Cookbook* and *A New Way of Eating*, both by Marilyn Diamond, from Warner Books.

High Fiber

As often as you desire, take advantage of The High-Fiber Cereal Lunch or Supper. We all love a bowl of cereal, and sometimes after a few days of fruit for breakfast, we find we're craving a cereal meal. Our solution: Have cereal for lunch or for supper! We especially enjoy *a blend* of various high-fiber cereals, mueslis, shredded wheats, and granolas with creamy vanilla soy milk—which we find highly digestible with grains. If you choose to use dairy milk, use a lactose-enriched product for better digestion. Have whole-grain toast, a whole-wheat bagel, or bread pudding with your cereal meal.

17

▼

The Jump-Start
for Quick Weight Loss

▼

Natural weight loss can sometimes be quite rapid and still be healthy. Frequently, when you embrace high-quality, natural foods three meals a day, the body responds enthusiastically by freeing up energy that not only is used for weight loss, but can also be felt as a positive surge in your daily routine. The FITONICS formula is an eating program you can enjoy for the rest of your life. What follows are some easy tools that can give you a jump-start for quick weight loss.

Making It Easy!

BREAKFAST

Every day you can take advantage of the quick and easy FIT-TONIC, the breakfast in a glass. Start with some fresh juice—for example, orange or apple, which we find to be the best bases for tonics. Add fresh or frozen bananas, strawberries, blueberries, peaches, or fresh apple, in short . . . any fruit you would like to include in your morning meal. Optional: For added sweetness, add a handful of raisins or a few pitted dates.

Finally, you also have the option of adding any number of whole food nutrient powders. The FIT-TONIC will give you enzymes and a true morning lift. It will cleanse your body and go a long way toward preventing constipation. We find that it fills us up so much, we aren't hungry for hours!

On occasion, when you feel like sitting down to some cereal in the morning, you can enjoy a FRUIT CEREAL, which can be made in a jiffy by shredding some apples, pears, and carrots; slicing bananas; and adding chopped nuts, dried fruits, or raisins. Pour apple juice or dairy or soy milk over your cereal, add a dusting of cinnamon . . . this is a winner if you love sweets!

A.M. SNACK

Have fruit or hot or iced herbal tea. If you wish to break a sugar habit, have some dates instead of a donut.

POWER LUNCH

This is the time for protein and vegetables, especially in the form of a salad, to give you the pickup and punch you're looking for during the afternoon. Proteins are stimulating and particularly satiating, so you'll find your midday protein meal keeps you satisfied and alert. You can have the protein of your choice—meat, poultry, fish, eggs, tofu, beans, or dairy mixed in with a salad. The raw salad vegetables break down on their own so your enzymes need work on only the protein.

We frequently use the concept of the High-Energy Super-Salad, a salad containing our protein and vegetable choices. The Chicken and Caesar Salad and Chef's Salad found on many restaurant menus are examples of this type of eating. We rev up the nutrient potential by adding plenty of sprouts, and in truth, after much trial and error, we can't offer a better solution or a more enjoyable and easier way to lose weight and cruise through our afternoon with plenty of energy.

Making the Super-Salad at home or having one put together in a restaurant is easy. To your favorite salad (or to the FITONICS House Salad, which is one of our favorites), you add whatever protein (or starch, for vegetarians) you are choosing for your lunch. In other words, you have two choices:

1. You can create this meal of salad ingredients such as lettuce, spinach, watercress, tomatoes, cucumber, radishes, and sprouts, and cooked vegetables such as zucchini, broccoli, asparagus, and peas. You can add meat, poultry, fish, tofu, eggs, or cheese. Feel free to combine proteins, such as ham and cheese or tuna and egg salad.

2. If you are choosing the vegetarian option, you will be adding pasta, beans, potatoes, rice, or other vegetarian choices to your salad ingredients. Or, you will be having a salad with bread. In all cases, add plenty of sprouts to increase your enzyme intake.

We cannot encourage you enough to explore the Super-Salad concept during the first two weeks of your FITONICS adventure. It will accelerate weight loss and help you form the habit of feeling light and energized after lunch.

The guideline for high-energy sandwiches at lunch is: Start with whole-grain bread and lots of vegetarian ingredients. For fillings use avocado, grilled mushrooms and other grilled vegetables, roasted red peppers, hummus, tofu salad, and all the fresh vegetables—such as tomatoes, cucumbers, lettuce, spinach, and sprouts—that go well on sandwiches.

For a slightly more filling option, you can add cheese or a small amount of meat, but be careful about adding too much protein. During the weight-loss phase, it can definitely weigh down a sandwich and add unwanted weight to your body. Have veggieburgers or vegetable-and-cheese pizzas, and always try to accompany your sandwich with a salad.

▼

Can I Have Dressing on My Salad?

Yes, you absolutely can! But not *all* dressings will help in your desire to lose weight. Many are loaded with fat and sugar and a myriad of chemicals that you don't need when you're trying to do something good for yourself, like *eat a salad*.

We've shared with you our favorite recipe for a basic, delicious, and healthful salad dressing (see page 317), with some of its variations, in the FITONICS recipes. It contains extra-virgin olive oil, which Mediterranean cultures have shown us to be the highest quality, most heart-healthy oil you can use. We incorporate lots of garlic, which helps lower blood cholesterol. We use fresh lemon juice for its alkalinity or unpasteurized apple cider vinegar for its richness in potassium, which keeps your arteries nice and supple. For creaminess, you'll find us adding plain yogurt for the enzymes and friendly bacteria it contains that help keep the colon cleansed. This is an easy dressing to make. You simply whip it up with a fork or whisk in your salad bowl, before adding the greens. When you are dining out, salad dressings can be an obstacle, unless you are choosing a fine restaurant. Here are some solutions:

- Ask for olive oil and lemon juice.
- A truly refreshing option is to simply squeeze fresh lemon over your salad.
- Whatever dressing you are choosing, ask to have it served on the side, and *lightly* dip each bite of salad into it. *Lightly* means *barely touch the vegetables to the dressing!*
- If the restaurant is Southwestern or Mexican, have salsa on your salad instead of dressing.
- Add a few tablespoons of yogurt to your salad instead of dressing. For a heartier, but healthful, salad, add some cottage cheese, as well.
- Use mashed avocado, thinned with water and seasoned with lemon, for a dressing containing fats that carry with them their own digestive enzymes.

▲

P.M. SNACK

Refresh and add more enzymes with a big glass of fresh vegetable juice or herbal tea. If you're feeling hungry, have a few high-fiber crackers spread with fruit-sweetened jam or avocado. On occasion, have a sugar-free cookie with herbal tea.

SOOTHING SUPPER

We call it the "Guru's Bowl," and since it can literally be a "meal in a bowl," we find it to be the easiest meal of all: your starch-and-veggie meal. Snuggle up to a big bowl of pasta and vegetables or mashed potatoes and gravy, to which you have added some steamed carrots and peas or other green vegetable. Along with a healthy chunk of fresh whole-grain bread, you can enjoy a thick vegetable soup. For a real treat, add a healthy baked food.

For more rapid weight loss, make your evening meal a bowl of all the different vegetables you feel like eating and change the flavors by adding Chinese, Indian, or Southwestern sauces.

BEDTIME SNACK

For a good night's sleep: a banana.

SAMPLE MENU

DAY ONE

BREAKFAST
1/2 grapefruit or a slice of melon
The FIT-TONIC and ten extra sit-ups

A.M. SNACK
More fruit, dates, herbal tea

POWER LUNCH
Philly Cheese Steak Salad

OR

Grilled Portabello Mushroom Sandwich
with tomato and cucumber salad

P.M. SNACK
Fresh vegetable juice or high-fiber crackers
with avocado or fruit juice–sweetened jam

SOOTHING SUPPER
Yellow Split-Pea Soup with Yams and Tomatoes
Oatmeal Currant Scones

BEDTIME SNACK
Banana

SAMPLE MENU

DAY TWO

BREAKFAST
Fresh Orange Juice
Fruit Cereal

A.M. SNACK
Fresh Vegetable Juice

POWER LUNCH
Farmer's Chop Suey
Country Cream of Carrot Soup

P.M. SNACK
Sugar-Free Whole-Grain Cookie
Herbal Tea

SOOTHING SUPPER
Lasagna FITONICS
Hot Whole-Grain Bread

SAMPLE MENU

DAY THREE

∽ Y O U R   L I V E   F O O D   D A Y ∽

Juice all day long, every two hours

OR

Juice and fruit all day long

OR

Four TONICS during the day, at regular intervals

OR

BREAKFAST
Juice and Fruit Cereal

A.M. SNACK
More juice or a piece of fruit

CLEANSING LUNCH
Salad with Avocado

P.M. SNACK
Carrot Blush

CLEANSING DINNER
Fruit Platter or
Crudité Platter with Dip or
Steamed Vegetable Plate

A Word About the Live Food Day

There's no mystery to doing it. You simply reach for all the fresh food choices. You start your morning with a large glass of fresh juice, which you nurse, as if it were a meal. You can stay on fresh fruit and vegetable juices throughout the day, if you like, drinking up to sixteen ounces at a time . . . slowly. (See page 295 for juice recipes you may never have experienced. Although we do drink lots of juices, especially vegetable juices, we tend toward TONICS with our fruit juices to offset the high fruit sugar content and its rapid absorption. Vegetable juices, as well, are much lower in calories.) Or you can drink a delicious TONIC or have meals of fresh fruit or salad. Just make sure to eat only fresh, uncooked natural food all day long.

"Drink at least ten to twelve
8-ounce glasses of water per day.
The liver needs plenty of water to
convert body fat into energy."

—Diane Epstein and Kathleen Thompson,
Feeding On Dreams

According to results of a national survey reported in *Parade Magazine,* Sunday is "decision day" for dieters, and a whopping 95 percent launch their diets on Sunday or Monday.[1] We find, as well, that Sunday and Monday are our best Funday options. But in our case, we ignore the diet mentality and, instead, reach for health.

---

[1]"What America Eats." *Parade Magazine,* November 4, 1995, p. 4.

You may prefer Monday for Funday because it comes at the start of your week, after a weekend of recreation and activity, and it symbolizes a housecleaning that allows the rest of the week to proceed more smoothly. It's a personal choice. What is most important is that you do have a Funday, for cleansing or celebrating, as regularly as possible, every week.

Most of the greatest spiritual teachers throughout history have taught about the benefits of simple eating. This is your chance to experience what they have been talking about. The benefits will be more than you can ever imagine. When you choose to focus on fresh fruits and vegetables in their natural state, you are eating low on the food chain, close to Nature. This allows your body to bring itself into harmony with the vibrations of the Earth. Free of the stimulating effects of cooked food, you can literally feel the life force moving through you. The very willingness to care for the "temple" in this way brings rewards far beyond the physical.

18

▼

The Basic Shopping List

▼

Most of the items you will need for your FITONICS kitchen can be found in the supermarket. Some require an occasional trip to the natural food store. For hard-to-find ingredients, see the Resource Guide for mail-order options.

Apple cider vinegar—This is the only vinegar Natural Health pioneers and we recommend you use. This is truly a wonder food, but only if it is unpasteurized. Then it is rich in enzymes and readily absorbable potassium that keeps your arteries supple. You'll find many brands in the natural food stores; look for the cloudy particulates, called the "mother," which indicate that the vinegar is unprocessed. White vinegar comes from coal tar. It's not a food. All other vinegars are highly acidic.

Asian sauces, bottled—These are available in abundance in natural food stores in sugar-free, low-salt versions, and they are excellent to keep on hand to spice up a bowl of steamed vegetables.

Barbecue sauces—Recommended in *FIT FOR LIFE.* After all these years, Robbie's is still the finest.

Beans, dried or canned—Soak dried beans overnight, drain, and cook in fresh water for one to two hours. To save time, keep canned beans on hand.

Beans, canned refried—The vegetarian variety are healthiest.

Bragg's Liquid Aminos—A pure, nonfermented salt substitute made from water and soybeans. It contains all the eight essential amino acids and is an excellent addition to any live food meal.

Butter—A "natural" fat that we have been eating for thousands of years. Fat substitutes, including margarine, are recent innovations that our bodies don't recognize as good. They cause the dangerous free-radical buildup that leads to increased cancer risk. A little butter, now and then, is a satisfying option that can offset our tendency to overeat because the meal just "didn't do it" for us. Unsalted butter is fresher because salt is used as a preservative.

Cereals—Whole-grain high-fiber, containing *at least* 4 grams of fiber per serving.

Cheeses, all kinds—Especially goat cheeses for better digestibility.

Chips, baked—A wonderful alternative to fried chips, and a way to avoid hidden fat substitutes and their grisly side effects. Garden of Eatin' makes the best in four flavors.

Condiments, sugar-free—Mayonnaise, ketchup, and barbecue sauces are sugar-free in the natural food stores.

Curry—A pungent Indian spice that brings heat to food and warmth to the body. The best-flavored curries can be found at natural food and specialty shops. Simple vegetables and salads, spiced with curry, tend to come alive. When your food is spicy, rather than bland, you will eat less and feel more satisfied.

Dijon mustard—A basic salad dressing ingredient.

Fantastic Foods—Time-saving, whole-grain mixes, instant hummuses, soups, and tofu seasonings make healthful eating easier than ever. In supermarkets and natural food stores.

Fish and seafood—Orange roughy is one of the cleanest fish, coming from New Zealand. Canned tuna, especially white albacore packed in water, is a good option to keep on hand for your Super-Salads.

Fruits—All.

Fruits, frozen—A good alternative during the winter for TONIC additions.

Fruits, sun-dried—All. Avoid sulfur dioxide, used in drying, as it is caustic to the stomach.

Garlic—Keep plenty on hand in a garlic container. Do not store in the refrigerator, unless you live in a humid climate. Garlic kills bacteria in the body. It is a very important ingredient in the Super-Salad.

Ginger—Buy the whole root and store in the refrigerator. Use within a week to ensure freshness. Put ginger in your juices to settle the stomach. It was proven in the 1980s to be more effective than Dramamine for nausea. Ginger aids digestion and stimulates the production of saliva. It is an important ingredient in Indian and Asian cooking, where much starch is used and ptyalin in the saliva is required for starch digestion.

Grains, whole—Breads, brown rice, whole-wheat couscous, bulghur, millet, quinoa. The latter four are found in natural food stores.

Gravy Master—A handy gravy enhancer, available in supermarkets.

Herbal teas.

Herbs and spices—All. The nonirradiated brands found in health food and specialty stores have better flavor.

Meats: beef, pork, lamb—Buy lean cuts of beef and look for organic meats.

Milk, enzyme-enriched—When you use a whole product, you'll feel more satisfied and be less likely to binge. Just don't overuse. The added enzymes will make the milk more digestible, but we find soy milk to be an even better option, when available.

Nuts and seeds—All raw. You release the enzymes in nuts and seeds if you soak them for 30 minutes or more before using. Soaked nuts can be drained, allowed to dry, and then stored in the refrigerator in a covered container for several weeks without spoilage.

Oats and oat flour—Oatmeal is one of your *best* cereal options.

Olives—Greek, green, black, Italian, French . . . they all add flavor and interest to salads, fish, and chicken dishes. When choosing your fats, you will find olives are an excellent choice since they are a whole food, which makes the fats they contain more digestible.

Olive oil—Extra-virgin, first pressing only. This is the finest olive oil—and why would you want to put anything but the finest, highest-quality oil into your arteries? Olive oil is mostly a monounsaturated fat, which helps keep the arteries clean rather than clogged. The better it is, the better-tasting your food and the healthier your body.

Peppercorns—Freshly ground, these add so much more flavor to food than the pepper in shakers.

Poultry—Skinless, boneless chicken breasts are handy to keep on hand. Look for organic.

Salsas, bottled—These make great salad dressings, toppings for fish, or dips for chips and crudités.

Salt—Cut down; for a salt with no additives, use kosher salt.

Salt, seasoned—There are excellent varieties at the natural food stores that contain no chemicals.

Soy milk—Available in natural food stores in vanilla, plain, chocolate, and carob flavors. Plain is usually available in supermarkets. A new product on the market called Silk from White Wave is a delicious soy milk packaged in a milk carton. Available at most natural food stores; ask your grocer to stock it as well.

Sprouts—Alfalfa, leek, onion, clover, sunflower, buckwheat, and mung bean are all excellent salad and sandwich fillers. Sprouted beans such as chickpeas and adzuki beans, and sprouted grains such as wheat berries, are highly concentrated and should be used more sparingly and not combined at all with cooked foods.

Sweeteners—Date sugar, Sucanat, brown rice syrup, sorghum, barley malt. These are whole sweeteners that can be found in natural food stores.

Tahini—A Middle Eastern sesame butter used instead of dairy to add creaminess to dressings, sauces, dips, and soups. This product is high in protein and calcium and is available in supermarkets and natural food stores.

Tamari—Wheat-free fermented soy sauce.

Tofu—This highly digestible alkaline source of protein is well-known for its cholesterol-reducing properties. As well as being rich in protein, such soy products also provide a rich source of calcium. It is easy to substitute tofu for chicken or cheese in many recipes.

Tomatoes—Canned whole, diced, and puréed for adding to soups and sauces. Use in moderation. Canned tomatoes are extremely acid.

Turmeric—The yellow East Indian spice that gives curry dishes their distinctive color.

Vegetables—All.

Vegetables, frozen—Peas, corn, lima beans, spinach, and artichoke hearts are among the most useful for adding to salads and soups. Other vegetables are better fresh whenever possible.

Whole-wheat pastry flour.

Yogurt—A basic salad dressing ingredient, topping for soup, base for creamy sauces, and excellent accompaniment to fruit.

PART FIVE

FITONICS™

RECIPES FOR LIFE!

FRUIT MEALS

A N D

FUNDAY RECIPES

This is your day to cleanse, energize,
and give your body a break from all the cooked food
you normally eat.

▼

If you choose to cleanse, you may do so by drinking
only fresh juices or tonics every two to three hours or
by eating only live food—fresh fruits and vegetables
in the form of salads, fruit plates, or crudité dips.

▼

If you make it through the whole day on fruit,
vegetables, or juice and crave something warm at
night, have lightly steamed vegetables.

Juice Works!

Fresh juices cleanse and nourish the body. They are the perfect basis for the fruit and whole food vegetable tonics you will have the option to drink as part of the FITONICS FORMULA. There are several juices or juice blends we recommend for maximum benefit. You can either make them yourself with a fruit or vegetable juicer or you can buy them from one of the increasingly accessible fresh juice stands.

As you drink these juices, it is imperative to remember that they are a *food*, not a beverage. DRINK THEM SLOWLY. Allow them to mix with the saliva in your mouth so your body has a chance to break them down and extract the nutrients. If you feel that fruit juices are overly concentrated in sugars for you, dilute them 50 percent with water to receive the cleansing benefits and focus, especially, on vegetable juices. These juices can be your first choice on any Live Food Day.

෨

Orange Sunshine

Pure orange juice, and that's what it is, a glass of liquid light.

෨

Grapefruit

Lower in sugar than orange, highly alkalinizing,
will lower blood cholesterol.

Tangerine or Tangelo

Few people realize how delicious the juices from these fruits can be, and frequently, in season, they will be even more affordable than oranges.

Apple Zinger

6 apples
Juice of ½ lemon
1 one-inch piece of fresh ginger (or more to taste)*

Carrot Blush

7 carrots
1 small beet
2 apples
1 one-inch piece fresh ginger (optional)*

---

*Ginger increases circulation to the stomach, thus enhancing digestion.

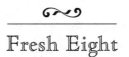

Fresh Eight

4 carrots
2 stalks of celery
Handful of parsley
1 small beet
2 tomatoes
1 red bell pepper
^{1}/₂ cucumber
2 cups alfalfa, clover, or sunflower sprouts
Optional: 2 cloves garlic, dash of cayenne

Melon Cleanse

^{1}/₂ small watermelon, including the green rind and seeds*
(for extra sweetness, add ^{1}/₂ peeled cantaloupe)

---

*The rind of watermelon contains needed nutrients, including chlorophyll, which helps detoxify the body and counteracts acidity. Without the rind, melon juice is mostly sugar. With the rind, the taste is actually enhanced.

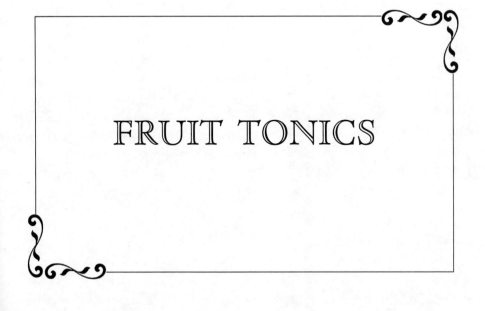

FRUIT TONICS

᠆᠊᠊

The Fit‑Tonic

5 MINUTES

2 cups fresh orange or apple juice
1 banana
Handful of raisins or pitted dates
1 heaping Tbs. green supernutrient formula*

1. Blend all ingredients until smooth and creamy. If you are adding powder, blend at least 30 seconds to thoroughly combine.

SERVES 2

᠆᠊᠊

Fit‑Tonic Plus

5 MINUTES

This is the basic cleansing tonic. Apples, bananas, and oranges are always available. If your fruit isn't sweet enough, blend in 1 or 2 dates or a handful of raisins.

2 cups fresh orange or apple juice
2 bananas
1 peeled navel orange or one quartered apple, peach, or
pear, seeded
Handful of raisins or pitted dates
1 Tbs. green supernutrient powder or protein meal
substitute*

---

*This might include spirulina, chlorella, blue-green algae, bee pollen, wheat grass, barley, or green lecithin. In addition to being rich in a wide range of nutrients, the green foods supply chlorophyll, which works like sunshine and carries oxygen to your body. Bee pollen supplies a wide variety of nutrients. Lecithin helps digest fat in the body. Just as mold thrive under rocks in the dark of the forest, in the dark corners of your body, ill health can take hold. The green nutrients let "the light" in. Ill health cannot grow in an oxygen-rich body. These whole food supplements are nutrient-dense, cleansing, and available in natural food stores.

1. Peel orange with a knife to leave as much of the nutritious white pith as possible. Leave peel on apple for added fiber.

2. Blend fruit until smooth and creamy.

3. Add green supernutrient formula, spirulina, or a blend of other freshwater algaes.

SERVES 2

6~9

Peach Melba Tonic

3 MINUTES

A creamy, nourishing treat for kids of all ages.

1 cup low-fat or soy milk
1 banana (fresh or frozen)
1 large peach, or 1 cup frozen peach slices
$1/2$ cup whole-milk yogurt (plain)
1 Tbs. maple syrup (optional)

1. Liquefy in blender. Drink slowly. This is not a true liquid. There's plenty of whole food in the glass!

SERVES 1

6~9

Bananaberry Tonic

3 MINUTES

1 cup orange juice
1 banana
$1/2$ cup fresh or frozen blueberries
$1/2$ cup fresh or frozen strawberries
1 Tbs. supernutrient powder

1. Place ingredients in blender and process until frothy and smooth.

SERVES 1

⌒〜〇

Strawberry Cream Tonic

2 MINUTES

1 cup low-fat or soy milk
8 strawberries (fresh or frozen)
1 banana (fresh or frozen)
1 scoop egg white or soy protein powder

1. Blend all ingredients until smooth.

SERVES 1

Note: When there's a need for a little extra fuel for your muscles, especially for vegetarians, be aware that the protein powder is not enzyme enriched and that enzyme supplements would be relevant with this tonic.

⌒〜〇

Apple-Pear Pudding

5 MINUTES

A delicious fall fruit salad.

1 1/2 cups grated apple
1 1/2 cups finely grated pear
1/4 cup raisins
1/2 cup apple juice
2 Tbs. ground almonds
Cinnamon to taste
2 sliced bananas or persimmons

1. In a bowl, mix apples, pears, raisins, and apple juice.

2. Sprinkle with ground almonds and cinnamon. Fold in sliced banana or persimmon.

SERVES 2

Fruinola

5 MINUTES

Who says granola has to be made from grain?

2 large crisp apples, peeled and cored
1 Tbs. currants
2 Tbs. shredded coconut (optional)
$^1/_4$ cup dried figs
$^1/_4$ cup coarsely ground almonds or sunflower seeds
2 tsp. maple syrup (optional)
$^1/_2$ tsp. ground cinnamon
$^1/_4$ cup fresh apple juice

1. Place the apples and currants in a food processor and coarsely grind.

2. Combine the apple mixture with the coconut, figs, almonds, maple syrup, cinnamon, and apple juice. Mix well.

SERVES 2

Note: For a more building meal, pour soy milk, rice milk, or low-fat milk over your "cereal."

Layers of Fruit with Compote

A nourishing, highly cleansing breakfast, lunch, or dinner, especially fueling in cool weather.

Compote

$^1/_2$ cup dried figs
$^1/_2$ cup dried apricots
$^1/_2$ cup dried pitted prunes
$^1/_2$ cup raisins

Fruit

2 bananas, thinly sliced
1 kiwi, peeled and sliced into thin rounds
1 pear, quartered, cored, peeled, and thinly sliced
8 strawberries, thinly sliced, or one peeled and sliced
   orange

1. Rehydrate dried fruit in 2 cups water overnight or for several hours.

2. Slice fruit in layers in shallow serving dish.

3. Spoon fruit into bowls, maintaining layers. Top with spoonfuls of compote and juice.

SERVES 4

Fresh Fuji Applesauce

10 MINUTES

Fuji apples have a special flavor and crispiness that you owe it to yourself to try!

1 large or 2 small Fuji apples, diced, unpeeled
2 tsp. maple syrup
$1/4$ tsp. cinnamon, or to taste
Dash nutmeg, or to taste
Dash cardamom, or to taste
2 Tbs. raisins
$1/4$ cup orange or apple juice

1. Combine all ingredients in blender or food processor and process until smooth.

SERVES 1

৬~৩

FITONICS Fruit Salad

5 MINUTES

This is our variation of Dr. Walker's favorite breakfast.
Remember, he lived to be 106!

2 ripe bananas, sliced thin or mashed
2 or 3 Tbs. carrot pulp or grated carrot
3 tsp. soaked raisins
1 apple, grated
1 Tbs. finely ground raw almonds or pecans (optional)*
$^1/_2$ cup apple juice

1. In a bowl, layer ingredients in the order given above, repeating each layer twice.

2. Pour juice over top.

SERVES 1 TO 2

৬~৩

Lettuce Roll-Ups

This is one of the best keys to making it through a live food day! Have this innovative salad meal with 2 ears of sweet, fresh, raw corn[†] for a satisfying lunch or supper. Surround it with fruit meals and tonics and see how energetic and alive you feel the following day.

1 head romaine or salad bowl lettuce
1 avocado
1 tomato, diced
2 Tbs. red onion, diced
Sprouts, sprouts, sprouts!
$^1/_4$ tsp. chili powder or a dash of cayenne

---

*Remember, to make nuts enzymatically rich, soak them to initiate sprouting for at least 30 minutes. This converts fats to fatty acids and proteins to amino acids and makes nuts nutritious and more easily digestible, rather than fattening.

[†]Raw corn on the cob, when it is fresh and in season, is one of the key options you can add to your Fundays and live food meals. Its sweet, milky quality gives a feeling of satiety and it is an excellent fiber, as well.

1. Separate lettuce into individual leaves.

2. Mash avocado and combine with remaining ingredients.

3. Spoon onto lettuce leaves, roll up and munch.

6~9

Carrot-Currant Salad

10 MINUTES

6 medium carrots, peeled and finely grated
¹/₄ cup currants or raisins, or to taste
3 Tbs. lemon juice
2 Tbs. maple or brown rice syrup
¹/₂ cup low-fat yogurt
¹/₂ tsp. cinnamon

1. Combine grated carrots and currants.

2. Combine remaining ingredients. Pour over carrot mixture and mix well.

SERVES 3

6~9

Pear, Avocado, and Kiwi Salad with Orange

5 MINUTES

2 pears, peeled and cubed
3 kiwis, peeled and cubed
1 avocado, cubed
1 orange, peeled, quartered, and sliced
¹/₂ cup sunflower or alfalfa sprouts, chipped

1. Combine and toss.

SERVES 2

꿈

FITONICS Sprout Salad

Sprouts as the basis for a salad are so brimming with enzymes and nutrients that your need for food (fuel) is satisfied with only a moderate portion. In fact, be careful not to overeat! Serve with a glass of fresh carrot juice (or carrot blush), jicama sticks, red pepper strips, and sliced cucumber.

2 cups mung bean sprouts
2 cups mixed sprouts (alfalfa, clover, onion, leek, garlic,
    radish, adzuki, or pea)
1 cup sunflower, snow pea,* or buckwheat sprouts
1 cup slivered bok choy or Chinese cabbage
2 sheets shredded, toasted nori†
2 green onions, chopped
1/2 cup Creamy Tahini Dressing

1. Combine all salad ingredients in large bowl.

2. Add dressing, toss thoroughly, and allow to marinate 15–30 minutes before eating.

SERVES 2

Creamy Tahini Dressing

You can make a large quantity of this dressing and keep it on hand in the refrigerator. It's especially good and rich on Fundays or at any live food meal.

1/2 cup tahini
Juice of one lemon
1/2 clove garlic or 1/4 small onion
Dash of cayenne pepper
1/2 tsp. thyme, basil, or dill
1–2 Tbs. Bragg's Liquid Aminos or other salt substitute or
    seasoning
Water (to thin to desired consistency)

---

*Use only upper leafy portion; stems are stingy.
†A pressed seaweed, rich in vitamins and calcium. Available in Asian section of supermarket.

1. Blend all ingredients to liquify, adding water to thin to desired consistency.

YIELDS AT LEAST 1¹/₂ CUPS

❦

Sushi "Alive"

25 MINUTES

Here's a recipe from The American Vegetarian Cookbook* *which is loved by young and old alike.*

¹/₄ cup sesame seeds
¹/₂ cup raw cashews
³/₄ cup lentil sprouts
1 medium carrot
¹/₂ small green bell pepper
1 4-inch celery stalk
2 Tbs. olive oil
1 leaf Chinese cabbage
2 tsp. tamari
8 sheets toasted nori
1 large tomato, halved and thinly sliced
Alfalfa and sunflower seed sprouts

1. Place the sesame seeds, cashews, and lentil sprouts in a food processor and process until thick and mealy. Add the carrot, pepper, and celery and process until smooth. Add the olive oil, cabbage, and tamari and process until the cabbage is chopped but not liquefied. (The cabbage should add some texture to the mixture.)

2. Spread approximately ¹/₂ cup filling on the lower half of a sheet of nori. Add a line of sliced tomatoes and sprouts. Roll and eat immediately or wrap in plastic wrap and store until ready to use. (As the sushi sits, the nori becomes less crunchy.)

SERVES 8

The American Vegetarian Cookbook, Marilyn Diamond. New York: Warner Books, 1990.

∽

Sesame Red Cabbage

$^{1}/_{2}$ *head red cabbage*
1 zucchini (optional)
1 small red onion
$^{1}/_{4}$ *cup toasted sesame seeds*
Juice of 1 lemon
Bragg's Liquid Aminos to taste

1. Shred cabbage, zucchini, and onion.

2. Mix all ingredients together and marinate 2 hours. Chill.

SERVES 2 TO 4

∽

Stuffed Mushrooms Florentine

$^{1}/_{2}$ *lb. (fresh white) mushrooms, stems removed*
$^{1}/_{2}$ *lb. spinach, washed well*
1 $^{1}/_{2}$ tsp. dried dill
Pinch of nutmeg
Pinch of cayenne
1 Tbs. lemon juice
$^{1}/_{4}$ *cup Creamy Tahini Dressing*

1. Clean mushroom caps and set aside.

2. Break down a few spinach leaves at a time in a food processor, using the S blade.

3. When all the spinach is finely chopped, add remaining ingredients.

4. Stuff the mushrooms and serve.

SERVES 2 TO 4

৶৶

FITONICS
Fantastic Meal for Weight Loss

Take any vegetable salad you enjoy,
mix with steamed vegetables of your choice,
and roll in hot whole-wheat tortillas.
Use condiments, such as salsa or mustard.
Have two or three.
You'll feel great,
and YOU'LL LOSE WEIGHT!

৶৶

ALTERNATIVES TO THE FRUIT BREAKFAST

❧

Poached Eggs on Toast

In the pre-cereal era, our grandparents and great-grandparents started their days with real meals like this.

1 or 2 free-range or veggie-fed eggs
Whole-grain toast or English muffin
1 tsp. apple cider vinegar

1. Poach eggs in water to which 1 tsp. apple cider vinegar is added.

2. Remove eggs from water with a slotted spoon and place on toast. Serve with hot chamomile tea.

❧

Yogurt and Pita Bread

This is a traditional Middle Eastern breakfast.

$^{1}/_{2}$ cup lowfat or whole plain yogurt
1 hot pita bread or whole-wheat bagel
2 Tbs. olive oil (optional)

1. Dip bread in oil and yogurt. Follow with hot mint tea.

6~9

Oatmeal with Poached Pears

15 MINUTES

For cold days when fruit just won't warm you enough, have this for breakfast, lunch, or dinner. It's like eating cake! Have it with a glass of soy milk flavored with potassium-rich black strap molasses.

Oatmeal
2 firm pears
$^1/_4$ cup raisins
$^1/_2$ cup water
1 Tbs. maple syrup or date sugar
1 tsp. cinnamon
Whole or low-fat milk* or vanilla soy milk

1. Prepare oatmeal according to package directions.

2. Peel and cut pears into bite-size slices.

3. Place pears in saucepan with remaining ingredients (except for milk).

4. Bring to boil, reduce heat to medium-low, and simmer, uncovered, for 5 minutes, testing and removing from heat when pears are tender. (Do not overcook to the point that pears break down.)

5. Spoon over hot oatmeal. Add 1 to 2 Tbs. milk or soy milk.

SERVES 2

*Try lactase-enriched milk for greater digestibility.

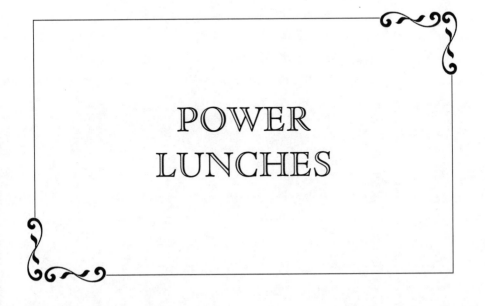

POWER
LUNCHES

⁓

FITONICS House Salad

10 MINUTES

A "house salad" consists of your favorite combination of vegetables and other ingredients. Our favorite is:

4 cups chopped spinach
1 diced tomato
2 cups steamed, sliced zucchini
1 cup alfalfa sprouts
8 Greek olives
^{1}/3 cup feta cheese (optional)
2 Tbs. minced cilantro or basil

Combine and toss with FITONICS dressing.

⁓

FITONICS Dressing*

3 MINUTES

Dr. N. W. Walker, the noted author of twelve books and the creator of the Norwalk Juicer, lived healthfully to the age of 106, died peacefully in his sleep, and recommended apple cider vinegar as the healthiest vinegar we can use. This is the basic dressing for any salad you wish to put together.

2 Tbs. olive oil
1 Tbs. water or broth
1 ^{1}/2 Tbs. lemon juice
1 tsp. apple cider vinegar (optional)
^{1}/4 cup whole or low-fat plain yogurt or buttermilk
^{1}/4 tsp. Dijon mustard
1 clove garlic, pressed

―――――

*Pour this dressing over any combination of greens for a basic green salad.

1. In a small bowl, whisk all ingredients. Pour over salad, or measure and whisk all ingredients directly into a large salad bowl and then add salad ingredients.

YIELDS $^1/_2$ CUP

6~9

Italian Salad

30 MINUTES

2 medium zucchini, sliced
$^1/_2$ lb. green beans, cut into one-and-a-half-inch
    segments
2 Roma tomatoes, sliced
1 cup chopped sunflower sprouts (optional)
$^1/_4$ cup thinly sliced red onion
6 cups mesclun with arugula
$^1/_4$ cup pitted Kalamata olives

Dressing

3 Tbs. olive oil
1 Tbs. fresh lemon juice
1 clove pressed garlic
$^1/_2$ tsp. Dijon mustard
Sea salt and pepper to taste

1. Steam zucchini until tender and bright green.

2. Boil green beans in an open pot for 10 minutes, or until bright and tender. Set aside.

3. Whisk dressing ingredients in the bottom of salad bowl until creamy. Add all the salad ingredients to the bowl and toss well.

SERVES 3

⟡

High-Energy Philly Cheese Steak Salad
30 MINUTES AFTER MARINATING

1 small flank steak (approximately ¹/₂ lb.)

Marinade

¹/₂ cup red wine
1 tsp. honey
2 cloves crushed garlic
Juice of one orange

Salad

4 cups assorted greens
2 cups alfalfa, clover, or spicy sprouts
¹/₂ cup slivered red onion
1 medium tomato, thinly sliced (optional)
¹/₂ cup shredded mozzarella cheese

Dressing

1 Tbs. olive oil
2 tsp. apple cider vinegar
1 tsp. lemon juice
1 tsp. tomato paste
1 tsp. Dijon mustard
2 cloves garlic, pressed
1 Tbs. water
Salt and pepper to taste

1. Marinate steak for 1 to several hours. Pan grill, 4 minutes per side. Slice paper-thin.

2. Combine steak and salad ingredients. Combine dressing and pour over salad. Toss well.

SERVES 2

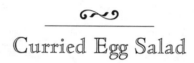

Curried Egg Salad

15 MINUTES

Serve with Caesar Salad and sliced tomatoes for a power-packed lunch.

4 hard-boiled eggs, grated, or $^{1}/_{2}$ lb. firm tofu, mashed
2 Tbs. mayonnaise
2 minced green onions
$^{1}/_{2}$ tsp. curry powder
$^{1}/_{4}$ tsp. cumin
$^{1}/_{4}$ tsp. coriander
$^{1}/_{4}$ tsp. turmeric (if you are using tofu)
Sea salt and pepper to taste

1. Combine and mix well.

SERVES 2

Caesar Salad

10 MINUTES

1 head romaine lettuce, washed and dried

Dressing

2 Tbs. olive oil
2 Tbs. water
$1^{1}/_{2}$ Tbs. lemon juice
1 tsp. apple cider vinegar
1 medium clove garlic, pressed
$^{1}/_{4}$–$^{1}/_{2}$ tsp. Dijon mustard
3 Tbs. buttermilk or yogurt
Freshly ground pepper to taste
2 Tbs. Parmesan cheese

1. Whisk all dressing ingredients but Parmesan together in a salad bowl. Add romaine, cut into bite-size pieces. Add Parmesan. Toss well. Season with pepper to taste.

SERVES 2 TO 3

All-American Chef's Salad

15 MINUTES

In a pinch, for a power lunch, you can find one of these just about anywhere.

¹/₂ head iceberg lettuce, chopped
1 oz. cheddar cheese, sliced into strips
1 oz. Swiss cheese, sliced into strips
1 oz. turkey, sliced into strips
1 oz. ham or roast beef, sliced into strips
1 tomato, sliced into wedges
1 hard-boiled egg, chopped
2 Tbs. sliced black olives

1. Combine all ingredients and toss lightly

Thousand Island Dressing

2 Tbs. sour cream
2 Tbs. mayonnaise
3 Tbs. ketchup
¹/₄ cup grated dill pickle

1. Combine and drizzle over salad.

SERVES 2

⌒〜♀

Shrimp Salad with Peas

20 MINUTES

1 1/2 lb. steamed shrimp
2 cups petite peas, cooked
1/4 cup chopped green onions
1/4 cup chopped parsley

Dressing

1/4 cup low-fat or whole mayonnaise
1/4 cup yogurt
1/2 tsp. curry powder
1/4 tsp. cumin
Sea salt and pepper to taste

1. Coarsely chop the shrimp. Place it in a mixing bowl with the peas, green onions, and parsley.

2. Combine mayonnaise, yogurt, curry, cumin, salt, and pepper in a small mixing bowl. Toss into shrimp and mix well to combine. Serve on a bed of greens with steamed zucchini and sliced tomatoes.

SERVES 3

⌒〜♀

Farmer's Chop Suey

20 MINUTES

This salad nicely complements artichokes for lunch or dinner.

2 cups chopped romaine lettuce
2 cups chopped iceberg lettuce
2 cups assorted sprouts
2 tomatoes, diced
1 cucumber, diced

2 *green onions, sliced*
6 *radishes, sliced*
¹/₂ cup sour cream
1 cup cottage cheese
1 tsp. apple cider vinegar
Salt and pepper to taste

1. Combine all vegetables in a large bowl. Mix together sour cream, cottage cheese, and vinegar in small bowl. Add salt and pepper to taste. Pour over salad, and mix thoroughly.

SERVES 2 TO 3

༒

Thai Chicken Salad

1 HOUR

If you are using cooked chicken, this is an easy 30-minute meal. Otherwise, add 25 minutes to cook chicken breasts. Serve with hot or iced green tea.

2 *chicken breast halves*
4 *cups shredded spinach, stems removed*
4 *cups bean sprouts*
2 *cups chopped snow peas*
1 *cup daikon matchsticks**
¹/₂ cup chopped cilantro
¹/₂ cup slivered green basil
¹/₄ cup finely sliced green onion
¹/₄ cup thinly sliced red onion
2 *navel oranges, peeled with a knife and cut into half-*
   inch segments

---

*Daikon is a large, long white radish used by the Japanese to help dissolve animal fat deposits in the body.

Dressing

2 Tbs. olive oil
1 Tbs. apple cider vinegar
2 Tbs. orange juice
1 tsp. powdered beef broth
3 Tbs. garlic-flavored teriyaki sauce
1 tsp. Szechwan sauce
2 cloves garlic, pressed
1 one-inch piece of ginger, pressed
2 Tbs. mirin or cooking sherry
2 Tbs. orange juice

Topping

$^1/_4$ cup finely chopped green onion tops

1. Place chicken breasts in a medium saucepan. Cover with water. Add 2 cloves garlic, $^1/_2$ onion, and 1 chopped stalk of celery. Bring to a boil. Cover and simmer 25 minutes or until tender. Drain and cool. (Save and freeze the broth to use in the future.)

2. Prepare all vegetables according to directions. Cut daikon into matchsticks by slicing in $^1/_8$-inch rounds, stacking rounds, and cutting into fine sticks.

3. Whisk all dressing ingredients together in the bottom of a large glass salad bowl.

4. Cut chicken into thin slivers.

5. Toss all vegetables and chicken in dressing. Spoon onto large glass plates. Top with chopped greens from green onions.

SERVES 3

❦

Kids' Salad with Three-Cheese Dressing

This is a basic salad both younger children and teenagers enjoy. The teenagers, especially boys, go for the onions. Children seem to prefer hothouse cucumbers because they are seedless.

2 cups iceberg lettuce, finely chopped
2 cups spinach, finely chopped
1 large tomato, halved and thinly sliced
1/2 medium hothouse cucumber, cut in quarters lengthwise and cubed
1/4 cup sliced red onion (optional)
1/2 cup alfalfa sprouts

Dressing

1/3 cup plain yogurt
2 Tbs. cottage cheese
2 Tbs. Parmesan cheese
2 Tbs. crumbled jack or cheddar cheese
2 tsp. apple cider vinegar
Spike to taste
1 clove garlic, pressed (optional)
2 Tbs. water
1/2 tsp. powdered vegetable or chicken broth

1. Combine dressing ingredients in large bowl.

2. Add chopped vegetables and sprouts.

3. Stir well.

SERVES 3 TO 4

ᕙᕗ

Veggie Deluxe Sandwich
with Carrot Chips

10 MINUTES

2 slices lightly toasted whole-grain bread
Tomatoes, very thinly sliced
Cucumber, thinly sliced
Roasted red peppers (available in jars)
Spinach leaves
Alfalfa sprouts
Avocado, thinly sliced
1–2 slices muenster or Swiss cheese (optional)*
Dijon mustard
Carrots

1. For carrot chips, slice carrots in thin diagonals.

SERVES 1

ᕙᕗ

Grilled Portabello Mushroom Sandwich

30 MINUTES AFTER MARINATING

A delicious complement to a steamy, hot bowl of soup.

4 large portabello mushrooms
2 Tbs. olive oil
1 tsp. minced garlic
2 Tbs. teriyaki sauce
1 Tbs. Szechwan sauce (optional)
4 Tbs. mayonnaise
4 tsp. Dijon mustard

---

*If you're craving cheese on your sandwich, know that all the raw, enzyme-rich vegetables will help make that option more digestible.

$^1/_2$ tsp. crushed garlic
2 slices sourdough olive bread or whole-grain bread
Thick slices fresh mozzarella cheese (optional)
Roasted yellow pepper halves
Thin-sliced red onion
Thin slices tomato
Sprigs of arugula

1. Marinate mushroom caps in mixture of olive oil, garlic, and teriyaki in the refrigerator for 30 minutes to several hours. Place on broiler pan and broil 15 minutes or until tender.

2. Mix together mayonnaise, mustard, and garlic.

3. Lightly toast bread. Place cheese on four of the slices and place under the broiler until cheese is melted. Top with mushroom, yellow pepper, onion, tomato, and arugula. Spread remaining slices with mayonnaise spread and use to top sandwich.

SERVES 4

ᕼᕽᕽ

Deli-Style Diet Plate

10 MINUTES

This is an easy and affordable Power Lunch solution.

1 lean beef hamburger, turkey burger, or veggie burger
1 sliced tomato
4 oz. cottage cheese
1 kosher pickle
8 oz. coleslaw

SERVES 1

◌~◌

Hummus

15 MINUTES

*A high-protein, high-fiber, Middle Eastern dip used
as a replacement for many dips and spreads.*

2 large cloves garlic
1 17-oz. can garbanzo beans, drained
$^1/_3$ cup tahini
$^1/_4$–$^1/_2$ cup water (for desired consistency)
Juice of 1 lemon

1. With food processor running, drop garlic through feed
tube to mince.

2. Add remaining ingredients and process until smooth.
Serve as a dip for crudités or as a spread for sandwiches.

YIELDS APPROXIMATELY 2 CUPS

◌~◌

Artichokes with Creamy Garlic Dip

1 HOUR

*A great accompaniment to salad, protein, or grain,
for lunch or supper.*

2 artichokes, stems and thorns trimmed, darkened outer
    leaves removed
2 cloves garlic, halved
1 bay leaf

Dip

2 Tbs. yogurt
1 Tbs. mayonnaise
1 tsp. Dijon mustard

2 tsp. lemon juice
2 cloves garlic, pressed

1. Place artichokes in steamer. Put halved garlic cloves and bay leaf in steaming water. Cover, bring to a boil, and steam over medium heat for 35 to 45 minutes, or until an artichoke leaf can be removed easily.

2. Whisk together dip ingredients. Serve with hot or cold artichokes.

SERVES 2

ᏜᎾ

Spinach Frittata

30 MINUTES

Serve with a basic green salad with FITONICS Dressing.

1 onion, minced
1 tsp. olive oil
1 12-oz. package frozen spinach, defrosted
8 oz. frozen corn, defrosted
3 eggs or 6 egg whites
1 cup whole or low-fat milk
¹/₄ cup grated Parmesan cheese
Sea salt and freshly ground black pepper to taste

1. Preheat oven to 375°.

2. In a medium skillet, sauté onion in olive oil about 5 minutes, until softened.

3. Drain the liquid from spinach and corn and discard. Add vegetables to onion and continue cooking 1 minute.

4. In a small bowl, beat eggs, milk, Parmesan, salt, and pepper until smooth. Pour into skillet and place in oven for 20 minutes or until set.

SERVES 3

~~~~~~~~~~~

Baked Fish Fillets Provencale

30 MINUTES

The vegetables and seasonings can be combined with the fish several hours before cooling. Cover and refrigerate until you are ready to bake.

> 1 lb. fish fillets (sole, grouper, snapper, etc.) or fish steaks
>   (swordfish, halibut, salmon)
> 1 large red or yellow tomato, sliced, or 1 cup canned
>   tomato chunks
> 1 bunch green onions, cut into one-inch segments
>   (1 cup)
> 1/3 cup chopped green or black olives (preferably Greek
>   style)
> Juice of 1 lemon
> Pinch of thyme
> Freshly ground pepper
> Seasoned salt or sea salt to taste
> Olive oil (optional)

1. Preheat oven to 375°. Brush medium baking pan with olive oil.

2. Wash and dry fillets and place in pan. Cover with vegetables, olives, lemon juice, and seasonings. Drizzle a thin stream of olive oil over top, if desired.

3. Bake for 15 to 25 minutes or until fish flakes with fork.

SERVES 3

oɔ

Oven-Roasted Herb-Crusted Chicken

50 MINUTES

This is one that's sure to please your kids. Double the recipe and keep on hand to toss into Power Lunch salads.

4 chicken thighs
4 chicken legs
$^1/_3$ cup butter
1 tsp. onion powder
1 tsp. garlic powder
$^1/_4$ tsp. paprika
$^1/_2$ tsp. thyme
$^1/_2$ tsp. chervil
Seasoned salt to taste
Fresh ground pepper to taste

1. Remove skin and fat. Wash chicken and pat dry with paper towels.

2. Dot with butter.

3. Dust with remaining seasonings. Bake at 375° for 45 minutes.

SERVES 4

⌒⌀⌒

Zucchini Pancakes with Yogurt

30 MINUTES

1 large or 4 small zucchini, trimmed (approximately $^3/_4$
   lb.)
3 Tbs. grated onion
$^1/_4$ cup Parmesan cheese (optional)
2 eggs or 3 egg whites
$^1/_2$ cup whole or low-fat milk or soy milk
Dash of hot pepper sauce
$^1/_2$ cup whole-wheat pastry flour
1 tsp. baking powder
Salt and pepper to taste
1 Tbs. olive oil
1 cup nonfat plain yogurt

1. Grate zucchini on medium-fine grater and place in colander. Thoroughly squeeze water from zucchini and place in medium bowl. Add grated onion, Parmesan, eggs, milk and pepper sauce.

2. Add flour and baking powder and mix thoroughly with fork. Season mixture with salt and pepper to taste.

3. Brush nonstick skillet with olive oil. Drop zucchini batter by heaping tablespoons on hot skillet. Fry until brown on both sides. Serve topped with yogurt.

SERVES 3 TO 4

༄

Spicy Turkey Loaf

1 HOUR AND 15 MINUTES

Serve with an Italian salad for a satisfying Power Lunch.

1 lb. ground turkey
2 Italian-style turkey sausages
2 Tbs. tomato paste
3 Tbs. ketchup
1 small onion, minced
2 cloves garlic, pressed
3 Tbs. applesauce*
1 egg or 2 egg whites
2 slice whole-grain bread, moistened and crumbled

1. Combine all ingredients and mix thoroughly. Form into an oval loaf and place in a shallow Pyrex dish. Bake at 350° for 1 hour or 325° for 45 minutes.

SERVES 4

Serve with Dijon Mustard Dip

3 Tbs. Dijon mustard
3 Tbs. yogurt
1 clove garlic, crushed

1. Combine and serve.

---

*Applesauce adds moisture to ground turkey.

⌒⌒

Now and Zen

20 MINUTES

This would be a traditional Japanese breakfast.

2 cups water
1 Tbs. mellow white or soy miso
1 cup firm tofu (cubed)
2 sheets nori, shredded
2 tsp. rice wine vinegar
1 tsp. hot sesame oil
Pinch of salt
1 cup sliced cucumber
1 tsp. black sesame seeds
$1/4$ lb. green soba
Ponzu sauce* or tamari sauce

1. Bring water to a boil. Remove $1/4$ cup boiling water from saucepan, add miso, and stir to a paste. Pour paste into boiled water, removed from heat. Stir in tofu and nori. Set aside.

2. Mix together rice wine vinegar and sesame oil, adding pinch of salt. Pour over cucumber. Sprinkle with sesame seeds.

3. Cook soba according to directions on package. Drain and cool. Pour Ponzu sauce over noodles.

4. Serve soup, cucumbers, and noodles in separate dishes.

SERVES 2

Note: Rice wine vinegar is traditional in Asian cooking and it is the one exception we make to apple cider vinegar.

---

*Available at natural food stores.

❦

Angel Hair Pasta Salad with Chicken and Spinach

30 MINUTES

This is a lovely buffet item, served hot or cold or at room temperature. For smaller quantities, cut the recipe exactly in half. This is also an example of using protein as a condiment.

1 lb. angel hair pasta
1 bunch spinach
4 green onions
1 sautéed or poached skinless, boneless chicken breast
1 Tbs. olive oil
1 Tbs. curry powder, or more, according to taste
1 tsp. turmeric
1 tsp. onion powder
1 tsp. powdered chicken or vegetable broth
$1/2$ cup water
1 cup nonfat plain yogurt
Seasoned salt and freshly ground pepper to taste

1. Cook pasta according to package directions for al dente.

2. While pasta cooks, thoroughly wash, dry, and chop spinach. Place in large bowl. Finely slice green onions and add to spinach.

3. Slice chicken breast into thin slivers.

4. Drain pasta, rinse briefly under cold water, drain well. Add warm pasta immediately to spinach-onion mixture, and toss with hands to wilt greens.

5. In pasta pot, heat olive oil and whisk in curry and turmeric. Cook one minute over low heat to release fragrance from spices. Add onion powder and powdered broth. Whisk in

water, remove from heat, and whisk in yogurt. Add chicken and combine well.

6. Pour sauce over pasta and greens, adjust seasonings, toss well.

SERVES 6 TO 8

૭~૭

Every Family's Favorite Chili

3 HOURS

A great Sunday project. It will fill your house with love while it fills your stomach with high-fiber food.

1/4 cup safflower or olive oil
1 1/2 lbs. organic chuck, cut into tiny cubes or "chili ground" (a coarse grind available on request from some butchers), or 1 1/2 lb. ground turkey, or 1 1/2 lbs. crumbled tofu
1 large onion, finely chopped
6 large cloves garlic, minced
2 Tbs. hot chili powder
2 Tbs. mild chili powder
1 Tbs. cumin
1 Tbs. paprika
1 tsp. oregano
2 14-oz. cans peeled and chunked tomatoes
1 14-oz. can chunky tomato sauce
1 cup bean broth from canned beans or water or more to taste, depending on how thick you like your chili
2 tsp. honey
1/4 cup dried minced onion
1 tsp. rock salt
1/2 cup fresh minced cilantro
1 jalapeño pepper, cut in half and seeded, or 1/2 tsp. cayenne (optional)

3 cups cooked red kidney beans, canned or fresh
Finely minced onion
Grated cheddar cheese (optional)

1. Heat oil in Dutch oven or covered soup pot. Add chuck, onion, and garlic and sauté, stirring frequently, until meat loses its color.

2. Add the chili powders, cumin, paprika, and oregano and cook for 5 minutes.

3. Stir in the tomatoes, tomato sauce, bean broth, honey, onion, salt, and cilantro. Add the jalapeño or cayenne for extra punch.

4. Bring to a boil, cover and simmer over low heat for 2 hours, stirring occasionally. During last 30 minutes stir in beans. Refrigerate overnight, if possible, to allow flavors to blend.

5. Serve with minced onion and cheddar cheese.

SERVES 6

SOOTHING
SUPPERS

૯~૭

Marilyn's Mashed Potatoes and Gravy

20 TO 25 MINUTES

A wonderful wintry-night supper. Serve with gravy and a mixture of steamed veggies.

4 baking potatoes, scrubbed and quartered (peel only if
    you don't think you need fiber)
3 cloves garlic, halved
1 small onion, halved
1 stalk celery, cut in chunks
1 bay leaf
6 peppercorns
4 Tbs. butter
$^1/_4$ cup yogurt
$^1/_3$ cup sour cream
Salt and pepper to taste

1. Put potatoes, garlic, onion, celery, bay leaf, and pepper-corns in a large saucepan. Cover with water. Bring to a boil.

2. Cover and simmer on low heat for 15 minutes or just until potatoes are tender (not mushy).

3. Remove potatoes to a large bowl with slotted spoon.

4. Melt butter, stir in yogurt and sour cream. Pour over potatoes. Mash with potato masher. Season to taste.

SERVES 3 TO 4

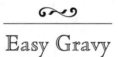

Easy Gravy

15 MINUTES

3 Tbs. canola or olive oil
3 Tbs. whole-wheat pastry flour
1½ cups potato broth
½ cup whole milk
Several drops Gravy Master*

1. Heat oil in medium Dutch oven. Add flour and whisk over medium heat until lightly browned. Stir in potato broth and milk slowly, whisking continuously to thicken. Season to taste.

SERVES 3 TO 4

Best Quick Sandwiches Ever

A great accompaniment with any soup.

2 slices toasted whole-grain bread
Almond butter to taste
Sliced banana to taste
Lots of clover or alfalfa sprouts
    OR
2 slices toasted whole-grain bread
Mayonnaise and/or mustard to taste
Sliced avocado
Sliced tomato
Lots of clover or alfalfa sprouts

---

*Available in all supermarkets.

൭ഛ

Country Cream of Carrot Soup
1 HOUR AND 10 MINUTES

One of our favorite recipes from Mom. Featured in FIT FOR LIFE II,
*this delicious soup can be served textured or blended to a smooth
cream. With the help of a food processor, it is a breeze to prepare.*

1 onion
2 ribs celery
1 Tbs. butter
6 medium carrots
$1/2$ cup parsley
Water
1 to 2 vegetable bouillon cubes
2 Tbs. cream (optional)
Seasoned salt or salt-free seasoning to taste

1. In a food processor, chop onion and celery. Melt butter
in a medium soup pot; add onion and celery and sauté. Meanwhile, coarsely grate carrots. Add to sautéing vegetables. Chop
parsley and add to vegetable mixture, stirring to combine.

2. Add water to cover vegetables by approximately $1/2$
inch. Add bouillon cubes and seasoned salt. Bring to a boil,
cover, and simmer for 1 hour.

3. For a richer soup stir in cream at end of cooking. Do
not return to a boil. For a carrot cream soup, blend soup and
add cream after blending. Serve hot or cold.

SERVES 4 TO 6

❦

Country-Style Miso Soup with Tofu, Noodles, and Vegetables

20 MINUTES

$1/2$ lb. Asian or buckwheat green noodles
4 cups water
$1/2$ lb. firm tofu, cut into bite-sized squares
2 large shiitake mushrooms, thinly sliced
2 cups bean sprouts
2 cups spinach leaves
3 heaping Tbs. mellow white miso
2 Tbs. soy sauce
4 sliced scallions, including greens from one scallion

1. Cook noodles according to package instructions. Drain, rinse well, and set aside.

2. Bring water to a boil. Add tofu, mushrooms, sprouts, and spinach. Cook about 2 minutes. Stir in noodles and remove from heat.

3. Remove half the water from the soup. Add miso and stir to dissolve to a thick paste. Pour miso mixture into soup. Do not reheat. Stir in soy sauce and green onions. Ladle into large bowls.

Quick Bean Soup

25 MINUTES

Serve with hot corn tortillas and avocado.

5 cups water
1 small onion, sliced
3 cloves garlic, minced, or 1 tsp. garlic powder
1 small carrot, cut in rounds
1 small zucchini, halved and sliced
1 1/2 cups broccoli or cauliflower florets
1 small tomato, chopped
1 Tbs. onion flakes
1 tsp. cumin
1 tsp. oregano
1/2 tsp. salt
Pepper to taste
1/2 tsp. chili powder (optional)
1 can pinto beans, drained
1 can refried beans
Shredded longhorn-style Colby cheese (optional)

1. Bring water to a boil. Add vegetables and seasonings. Simmer 10 minutes.

2. Stir in beans and simmer an additional 10 minutes. Adjust seasoning.

SERVES 4

⌒⌒

Creamy Soup of Petit Pois with Leeks

30 MINUTES

Serve with bread pudding. Yum!

6 cups water
2 celery ribs
1 large leek
1 small onion
3 cloves garlic
1 small potato
1 bag of frozen petit pois
3 Tbs. powdered chicken broth
1 Tbs. dried dill
1 Tbs. dried basil
Salt and freshly ground pepper to taste

Garnish

4 leaves romaine lettuce
$^1/_4$ sliced red onion

1. Bring water to a boil.

2. Slice celery. Cut leek in half lengthwise and slice. Place segments in a bowl of water to remove sand. Drain well. Chop onion and cut garlic in several pieces. Peel potato and coarsely chop. Add cut vegetables to boiling water. Add frozen peas and return to a boil.

3. Stir in powdered broth, dill, and basil. Cover and simmer soup over medium-low heat for 20 minutes, or until all vegetables are tender. Cool slightly and blend until creamy in several batches. Return soup to pot.

4. Chop romaine fine. Add with onion to soup. Return to a gentle boil. Adjust seasonings. Serve warm or chilled.

SERVES 5

⌒〜⌒

Hungarian Cabbage Soup

1 HOUR

Serve with Oatmeal-Currant Scones.

1 Tbs. olive oil
6 cups finely shredded red cabbage
1 large onion, chopped
1 large apple, peeled, and diced
3 large minced garlic cloves
1–2 tsp. caraway seeds, according to taste
2 14-oz. cans chopped or diced tomatoes, with juice
2 Tbs. apple cider vinegar
7 cups chicken stock
1 bay leaf
Salt and pepper to taste

1. In large saucepan, combine oil, cabbage, onion, apple, and garlic. Sauté for 10 minutes until vegetables are soft.

2. Stir in caraway seeds, tomatoes, vinegar, stock, and bay leaf.

3. Gently simmer 30 minutes.

4. Remove bay leaf. Season with salt and pepper.

SERVES 4 TO 6

〜

Yellow Split Pea Soup
with Yams and Tomatoes

A weekend recipe that will fill your home full of warmth and good cheer. Serve with Carrot Bran Muffins.

2 HOURS AND 30 MINUTES

1 Tbs. olive or safflower oil
2 cups onion, chopped
1/2 cup celery, chopped
2 Tbs. garlic, minced
1 tsp. garam marsala
1 tsp. cumin
2 tsp. coriander
2 cups yellow split-peas, rinsed and drained
4 cups vegetable stock
8 cups water
1 can peeled and diced tomatoes, with juice
4 bay leaves
1 Tbs. oregano
2 Tbs. minced dried onion
3 cups prebaked sweet potatoes or yams, peeled and
    diced
1 box frozen petite peas
1 bunch cilantro, chopped (1 cup)
1 tsp. salt
Freshly ground pepper

1. Put everything in a pot and cook the bajeebers out of it! Stir occasionally.

SERVES 8 TO 10

⌒∼⌒

Quick Tofu "Hot Pot"

A high-protein soup that will "go down" easily and give you a restful night's sleep.

10 MINUTES

2 cups chicken or vegetable broth
1 bunch chopped spinach
1/2 cup sliced daikon radish
4 green onions, sliced
1/2 lb. cubed tofu
1 8-oz. can stewed tomatoes, or 1 large fresh tomato, cut in chunks
1 large clove garlic, crushed
Tamari or Szechwan sauce to taste

1. Heat broth.

2. Stir in spinach, radish, and onions. Simmer briefly.

3. Add tofu and tomatoes. Heat through.

4. Stir in crushed garlic. Season with tamari to taste.

SERVES 1 TO 2

⟨⟩

Moroccan Vegetable Stew

45 MINUTES

1 medium onion, thinly sliced
1 medium red bell pepper, cut into half-inch strips and
   then in one-inch lengths
1 tsp. cinnamon
2 tsp. cumin
$1/4$ tsp. cayenne pepper
3 medium tomatoes, peeled, or 4 canned plum tomatoes
$1/2$ cup blended fresh tomatoes, or $1/2$ cup tomato juice
2 Tbs. lime or lemon juice
4 strands saffron
4 small new potatoes, cut in quarters (approx. 3 cups;
   optional)
3 medium carrots, sliced in quarter-inch chunks (approx.
   2 cups)
1 15-oz. can cooked chickpeas
1 tsp. salt
6 cups cooked couscous

1. In large pot, heat the onion and red pepper over medium heat. Add cinnamon, cumin, and cayenne and cook, stirring occasionally, for 5 minutes or until vegetables are soft.

2. Add a tablespoon or two of water, if needed. Add the tomatoes and juice and break up the tomatoes with a large spoon. Add the lime juice, saffron, potatoes, carrots, and chickpeas.

3. Increase to moderately high heat and bring to a boil. Reduce the heat to moderately low, cover, and simmer until the vegetables are tender, 10 to 15 minutes. Season with salt. Allow to sit for flavors to blend. Serve with couscous.

SERVES 3 TO 4

Curried Vegetables and Tofu

45 MINUTES

1 ear corn
1 small onion
1 small head cauliflower
1 bunch green onions
$^{1}/_{2}$ lb. tofu
1 medium tomato
$^{1}/_{2}$ tsp. safflower oil
1 tsp. black mustard seeds
    (optional)

2 tsp. curry powder
1 tsp. cumin
1 tsp. coriander
$^{1}/_{2}$ tsp. garam masala
$^{1}/_{2}$ tsp. ginger
$^{1}/_{2}$ tsp. salt
$^{1}/_{2}$ cup chopped cilantro
$^{3}/_{4}$ cup yogurt
1 tsp. lime juice

1. Cut corn from cob. Coarsely chop onion. Break cauliflower into florets. Slice green onions. Cut tofu into half-inch cubes. Cube tomato. Set aside.

2. Heat oil over medium heat in medium saucepan. Add mustard seeds and cover with lid for 15 seconds as seeds pop. Remove lid and stir in curry, cumin, coriander, garam masala, ginger, and salt.

3. Stir in corn, tofu, cauliflower, onion, green onion, cilantro, and tomato. Stir well. Add 2 tbs. water and stir. Cover and steam, stirring occasionally, for 25 minutes.

4. Remove lid and remove pan from heat. Stir in yogurt and lime juice.

SERVES 3

To Serve: Spoon over hot brown basmati rice or whole-wheat couscous. Top with yogurt and chutney.

ᏳᏒᎧ

Curried Linguine with Chicken and Broccoli

25 MINUTES

A hot version of the Angel Hair Pasta Salad using broccoli instead of spinach. Again, an example of protein as a condiment.

> ¹/₂ lb. linguine
> 4 cups broccoli florets
> 1 boneless, skinless chicken breast, sautéed or poached
> 1 tsp. olive or safflower oil
> 1 ¹/₂ tsp. curry powder
> 2 green onions, sliced
> 4 heaping Tbs. nonfat plain yogurt
> ¹/₂ tsp. seasoned salt

1. Cook linguine al dente according to package directions while you prepare other ingredients.

2. Steam broccoli until bright green and al dente, approximately 5 minutes. Remove from heat and set aside.

3. Cut chicken breast into thin slivers.

4. Drain pasta and set aside.

5. Using pot in which pasta was cooked, heat oil and add curry. Cook one minute, whisking continuously. Stir in green onion, whisk for 30 seconds. Stir in yogurt and remove from heat, whisking until smooth.

6. Add pasta, broccoli, and chicken to sauce in pot. Season with salt. Stir gently with a spatula or wooden spoon to combine.

SERVES 2, IN LARGE BOWLS, AS A ONE-DISH MEAL. PASS HOT BREAD, IF DESIRED.

⚬~❡

Spicy Avocado Spread

15 MINUTES

1 ripe avocado, peeled and seeded
2 Tbs. minced red onion
1 clove garlic, pressed
1/8 tsp. chili powder
1/8 tsp. cayenne pepper
2 tsp. water

1. Mash avocado with a fork. Whip in onion, garlic, spices, and water. Spread on hot or toasted whole-grain bread.

SERVES 3

⚬~❡

Artichoke Rice

15 MINUTES

A quick grain supper with salad. Delicious!

3/4 cup Minute brown rice
1 tsp. low-sodium tamari
1/2 box frozen artichokes

1. Prepare rice according to package directions.

2. Add tamari and chopped artichokes and an additional 1/4 cup water and steam over low heat for 10 to 15 minutes.

SERVES 1 TO 2

ᕫᕬᕬᕙ

Toasted Bean-and-Cheese "Burro"*

10 MINUTES

A traditional Southwestern high-fiber meal.

1 cup refried beans (freshly made or canned)
¹/₄–¹/₃ cup shredded longhorn-style Colby cheese
    (optional)
1 large flour tortilla (preferably whole wheat)

1. Heat skillet to medium. Heat beans in a small saucepan.

2. Place beans and cheese in center of tortilla. Fold in sides and roll tortilla, envelope style.

3. Place burro on hot skillet. Toast for 1 minute per side until lightly brown.

SERVES 1

Note: Serve with Mexican-style rice for a soothing supper.

ᕫᕬᕬᕙ

Mexican Rice

When you put rice to cook, add ¹/₄ cup minced onion,
¹/₂ tsp. garlic powder, and 1 tomato, chopped.

---

*A burro is a king-sized burrito made with a large tortilla.

Baked Beets and Vegetable Platter

20 MINUTES OR 1 HOUR AND 30 MINUTES

If you've never eaten a baked beet you deserve to treat yourself to this experience, but if you are short on time, simply heat whole canned beats on the stove for a few minutes.

6 medium beets
2 bunches beet greens
2 medium zucchini, sliced
1 lb. asparagus, trimmed
^{1}/4 cup olive oil
1 ^{1}/2 Tbs. apple cider vinegar
1 Tbs. soy sauce, or tamari
1 clove crushed garlic (optional)

1. Wash and trim beets of greens. Leave root end intact to avoid bleeding. Bake beets 1 to 1^1/2 hours at 350°, or until tender. Cool slightly and peel.

2. Steam beet greens and sliced zucchini separately. Boil asparagus in water to cover for 5 minutes, uncovered, or until bright green and al dente.

3. Slice or cube beets. Arrange on platter with zucchini, beet greens, and asparagus.

4. Whisk together oil, vinegar, soy sauce, *or* tamari and garlic. Drizzle over vegetables.

SERVES 4

⌒

Curried Spinach and Tofu

30 MINUTES

Try this fabulous vegetarian meal!

³/₄ lb. firm tofu
2 bunches fresh spinach, or 4 boxes frozen chopped
    spinach, thawed
1 bunch green onions
¹/₂ Tbs. safflower oil
1 tsp. curry
1 tsp. coriander
¹/₂ tsp. garam masala
¹/₂ tsp. salt
1 tsp. lime juice
¹/₂ cup thick whole or low-fat plain yogurt

1. Cut tofu in half-inch cubes. Finely chop spinach. Slice green onion. Set ingredients aside.

2. In Dutch sauté pan, heat oil, curry, coriander, and garam masala for 1 minute over medium-low heat until spices become aromatic.

3. Add onions and tofu. Sauté, stirring frequently, for 5 minutes. Add spinach, mix well, and cover. Allow to steam for 15 minutes, stirring occasionally. Remove lid. Stir in lime juice and yogurt and continue cooling and stirring until spinach is broken down to a creamy consistency.

4. Serve with Whole-Wheat Couscous. Top with yogurt and chutney.

SERVES 3

Quick Cabbage Borscht

40 MINUTES

1 Tbs. olive oil
1 medium onion, sliced
3 cups coarsely chopped cabbage
2 cloves garlic, chopped
1 stalk celery, sliced
1 carrot, cut in thin rounds
1 zucchini, sliced
1 small apple, peeled and cubed
1 14-oz. can crushed tomatoes
1 Tbs. minced, dried onion
2 vegetable or chicken bouillon cubes
6–8 cups water
1 tsp. dill
3 Tbs. lemon juice or apple cider vinegar
2 Tbs. honey
$1/4$ tsp. chili powder (optional)
Dash of cayenne pepper

1. Place olive oil and next seven ingredients in soup pot. Sauté briefly.

2. Stir in remaining ingredients.

3. Simmer 20 minutes. Serve with Date-Nut Bread with Orange Cream Cheese and a salad, if desired.

SERVES 6

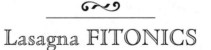

White Beans and Spinach in the Wok

A pleasing accompaniment to grilled chicken or lamb. this dish also can be a main course with corn on the cob and whole-wheat sourdough garlic bread. It is also a fabulous addition to pasta.

1 bunch fresh spinach, cleaned
2 tsp. olive oil
1 large clove garlic, crushed
1 can Great Northern beans, drained
1 small tomato, diced
Fresh ground white pepper

1. Place spinach, olive oil, and garlic in a heated wok. Stir to coat spinach with oil.

2. Add beans and stir to combine with spinach and heat through. Stir in diced tomato. Season with pepper.

SERVES 4

Lasagna FITONICS

1 HOUR AND 20 MINUTES

For entertaining or Sunday suppers, this nontraditional lasagna is a breeze to put together.

1 recipe Quick Bolognese Sauce
8 lasagna noodles
2 medium zucchini, sliced on diagonal
2 carrots, thinly sliced
1 Tbs. honey
1 tsp. basil
½ cup ricotta cheese

Quick Bolognese Sauce

30 MINUTES

Prepare this delicious sauce in 30 minutes with extra lean ground sirloin, ground turkey, crumbled firm tofu, or crumbled vegie-tofu or tempeh burgers.

1/4 cup extra virgin olive oil
6 large cloves garlic, minced
1 large onion, finely chopped
1 1/2 lbs. ground beef or turkey, or vegetarian substitutes
1 1/2 Tbs. tomato paste
1 8-oz. can tomato sauce
3 14-oz. cans Italian-style crushed tomatoes
1 Tbs. dried basil
1 tsp. dried oregano
1/4 tsp. red pepper flakes or cayenne to taste
2 tsp. powdered beef-flavored broth or 1 beef or chicken
    bouillon cube
Salt and pepper to taste

1. Heat oil, garlic, and onion in a large saucepan. Sauté over medium-low heat until transparent.

2. Break ground meat into saucepan and sauté until it loses color completely.

3. Add tomato paste, sauce, and crushed tomatoes. Stir in basil, oregano, pepper flakes, and broth or bouillon. Mix well.

4. Bring sauce to a boil, reduce heat, and simmer, uncovered, for 10 minutes. Season with salt and pepper.

YIELDS APPROXIMATELY 8 CUPS

5. As sauce is cooling, prepare vegetables. Steam zucchini lightly. Place carrots in water to cover with honey and basil. Cook, uncovered, until water is absorbed and carrots are tender.

6. Cook pasta until al dente.

To Assemble Lasagna:

7. Place several noodles, randomly folded, on three dinner plates. Top with layers of zucchini, carrots, and several dollops of ricotta, and, finally, ladle sauce over all.

SERVES 3

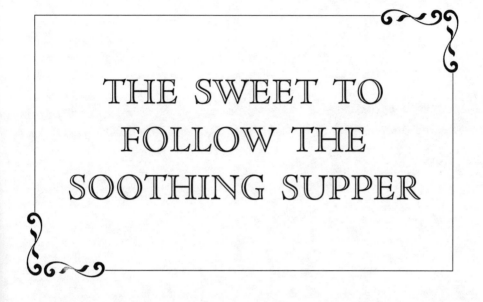

THE SWEET TO
FOLLOW THE
SOOTHING SUPPER

⟨⟩

Oatmeal-Currant Scones

30 MINUTES

1 cup orange juice
1 cup dried currants
1 cup all-purpose unbleached flour
1 cup oat flour
1 1/2 cups quick oats
1/4 cup dry sweetener
1 tsp. baking powder
1 tsp. baking soda
1 tsp. sea salt
1/4 cup sweet butter
2 cups buttermilk

1. Preheat oven to 375°.

2. In a small saucepan, bring orange juice to a boil and add currants. Remove from heat and set aside.

3. In large mixing bowl, combine flour, oats, sweetener, leavening, and sea salt. Cut in butter in tablespoon-size chunks. By hand, rub (or flake) butter into dry ingredients until mixture resembles coarse crumbs. Drain currants and add to flour mixture.

4. Add buttermilk all at once and stir with wooden spoon just until mixture binds together into a manageable dough. Transfer dough to a well-floured surface and knead about 10 times.

5. Line baking sheet with parchment paper and pull off one handful of dough at a time, dropping about 1¹/₂ inches apart on sheet. DO NOT ATTEMPT TO SHAPE OR FLATTEN SCONES.

6. Bake 20 minutes and cool on wire racks.

YIELDS 10–12 BISCUITS

$\sim$

Deluxe Fruit Plate

10 MINUTES

A great Soothing Supper when weight loss is on your mind.

Sliced melon (cantaloupe, watermelon, and/or
*   honeydew)*
Sliced bananas, oranges, apples, or pears
Grapes, berries, papaya, mangoes, plums, peaches
2 Tbs. unsweetened coconut
2 Tbs. raisins
1/2–1 cup fresh low-fat plain yogurt or cottage cheese

1. Choose 5 fruits. Top with coconut and raisins—and yogurt, for a slightly heavier, more filling meal.

SERVES 1

Note: This is the perfect meal when you want the cleansing benefits of fruit and a little something more.

Banana-Date Bread Pudding

45 MINUTES

3 cups whole-grain bread
1 cup mashed bananas
$^1/_2$ cup coarsely chopped pitted dates or raisins*
1 cup milk or soy milk
$^1/_4$ cup apple juice concentrate
2 egg whites or whole eggs
3 Tbs. butter, melted (optional)

1. Preheat oven to 375°.

2. Cut bread into one-and-a-half-inch cubes.

3. In a large bowl, combine remaining ingredients and mix well. Add bread cubes and soak until liquid has been absorbed (about 10 minutes).

4. Transfer to 9″ × 4″ (or equivalent) loaf pan or Pyrex dish. Bake 35 minutes. Slice and serve.

SERVES 6

---

*Chocolate chips can be substituted for the dates or raisins.

6~9

Date-Nut Bread
with Orange Cream Cheese

1 HOUR AND 15 MINUTES

4 cups wheat bran flakes
2 cups all-purpose unbleached flour
2 cups whole-wheat flour
3 Tbs. baking powder
1 1/2 tsp. salt
1 1/2 cups honey
1 cup molasses
2 cups buttermilk
4 eggs
1/2 cup melted butter
1/2 cup puréed dates
1/2 cup date chunks
1 cup mixed chopped nuts

1. Preheat oven to 375°. Butter and flour two loaf pans.

2. In a large mixing bowl, stir together dry ingredients.

3. In a separate bowl, combine wet ingredients, date pieces, and nuts. Fold wet ingredients into dry.

4. Divide batter between the two loaf pans and bake about 1 hour, or until a knife inserted in the center emerges clean.

Cream Cheese Spread

6 oz. soft cream cheese
1 Tbs. orange zest
2 Tbs. honey
Pinch of salt

1. Whip together to combine.

⧼⧽

Carrot Bran Muffins

30 MINUTES

1 1/2 cups bran flakes
3 Tbs. safflower oil
1/2 cup buttermilk
1 egg white
2 cups grated carrot
1 cup honey
1/2 cup crushed pineapple
1/2 cup raisins
2 cups whole-wheat pastry flour
2 tsp. baking powder
1 tsp. baking soda
1 tsp. cinnamon
1 Tbs. carob powder
1/2 tsp. sea salt

1. Preheat oven to 375°.

2. Combine bran flakes, oil, buttermilk, egg white, carrot, and honey in a large mixing bowl. Add crushed pineapple and raisins.

3. Stir together remaining ingredients and fold into carrot mixture. Mix well and spoon batter into 12 paper-lined muffin cups.

4. Bake 20 to 25 minutes, or until a toothpick inserted emerges clean.

YIELDS 12 MUFFINS

▼

Namasté

▼

Namasté.

Now, what does that mean? *Namasté* is an ancient Sanskrit word that means "I honor the Divine essence within you." Before you say, "Oh-oh, here we go with one more contemplate your navel and visualize yourself into Nirvana" message, we want you to know that what we mean by "Divine" is this great mystery, the principle of life that you embody.

We say *Namasté* because we truly do honor this life force. We honor it in ourselves, and we honor it in others, and it is our goal for you to do the same. By honoring the life force that flows from the Divine essence in each of us, we have no choice but to embrace a lifestyle that will make us healthy. So many of our society's troubles—even the epidemics of excess weight and disease—have come about because, as a culture, we have failed first, before anything else, to acknowledge and honor the Divine or life force within each and every one of us. Some of our greatest Transcendental philosophers, such as Emerson, Whitman, and Thoreau, talk to us about this life force, which they refer to as "the Soul."

Maybe you've heard what we're going to say now said in other ways, and we want to say it in terms that, we hope, will resonate and deepen your understanding of what constitutes your ultimate health:

You, dear friend, are a spiritual being, a Soul, with tools to make your human experience possible. What are those tools? They're your greatest resources: a healthy body and a healthy mind. Your journey as a spiritual being is through an intelligent, purposeful universe, and the life you lead is, in essence, a "school" at which you master the higher emotions and let go of those that bring you down. You are here for a reason. That reason is to embrace love, joy, peace, and health—in other words, all that leads to spiritual growth and evolution.

As Antoine de Saint-Exupéry stated in *Le Petit Prince*, "We must get to what is essential." Without what is essential, an appreciation—a reverence—for life, the higher awareness, the pursuit of health, is a vain mockery, an exercise in vanity, which can lead only to ultimate pain. How sad to see those who spend entire lifetimes focused in vanity on the body, only to watch in panic and emptiness its ultimate decay.

Without the essential reverence, there is no way to uncover the secret to health and lasting happiness. It is this very reverence for life that science and medicine have missed and continue to deny in the development of modern medical treatment. In their mechanistic worldview, they have sadly overlooked the biological life force, the Divine energy that animates all we see. That energy, nurtured and unleashed, can bring about more health and healing than costly technological innovation.

Great spiritual and philosophical sages—in every culture and tradition—have taught us that a reverence for life is the key to individual health and the advancement of society. So, in solving your health and weight-loss problems, we're suggesting that the place to start is with an unreserved connection to the life force within you. It emanates from your Soul in the same way that rays of light emanate from the sun. The more you fuel and nurture it, the more swiftly will you return to the health and normal weight that are your birthright.

From yoga, from the ancient Hebrews, and from other great spiritual traditions, for thousands of years has come the reminder that the body is merely our vehicle through life. We are taught to use the magical tool of the mind to access our own personal Divinity. It is said both body and mind serve the Soul as it strives to accomplish the missions of your life. This is now your opportunity.

You have, at your fingertips, the guidelines to make your body and your mind the vehicles you need to realize all the dreams of your Soul. Your *balance.* At this very moment, you can embrace the ancient human tradition of reverence for the Gift of Life that has so long eluded our culture.

You can have in your grasp the supreme balance of body, mind, and spirit that yields not only desired weight loss, not only radiant health, but also the sunny state of being that is your birthright. Life is not an accident, and your health and longevity are not accidental either.

We honor that life force within you, and we celebrate your readiness to do the same. Undeniably, LIFE IS WHAT YOU MAKE IT, and day by day, we will enjoy witnessing you grow stronger and more full of cheer as you develop the mental habits and physical behaviors that validate "what is essential." The validation that you will now be cultivating through FITONICS will activate, awaken, and ready your life force for healing and growth.

And therefore, until next we meet, we bid you FAREWELL . . . and . . .

Namasté.

Resource Guide

▼

Organic and Specialty Foods

JAFFEE BROTHERS NATURAL FOODS (since 1948)
P.O. Box 636
Valley Center, CA 92082-0636
619-749-1133
Fax: 619-749-1282

Organic dried fruits, peas and beans, seeds, grains and flour, whole-wheat pasta, nonwheat pasta, tomato products, dehydrated vegetables, nuts, nut butters, jams, oils, olives, condiments, baking needs, snacks and treats, herbal teas, coffee, soy milk powder, soaps, and shampoos.

DIAMOND ORGANICS
P.O. Box 2159
Freedom, CA 95019
800-922-2396
E-mail address: organics@diamond-organics.com

Organic fruit, salad greens, exotic mushrooms, fresh herbs and edible flowers, pastas and breads, vegetables, prepared meals, sprouts, roots and tubers, dried fruits and nuts, gift items. (This company ships fresh produce and meals overnight; orders must be placed by phone or fax.)

ROBBIE'S NATURAL PRODUCTS
1920 N. Lake Avenue, #108-182
Alta Dena, CA 91001

Sugar-free barbecue sauce, sweet-and-sour sauce, salsa, syrups, ketchup, garlic sauce, spaghetti sauce, Worcestershire sauce.

AMERICAN SPOON FOODS
P.O. Box 556
1688 Clarion Avenue
Petoskey, MI 49770-0566
800-222-5886
616-347-9030
Fax: 616-347-2512

Pure, unprocessed honeys and sugar-free fruit butters, jams, and jellies.

CINNABAR SPECIALTY FOODS
214 Frontier Drive
Prescott, AZ 86303
800-824-4563
602-778-3687

Chutneys and East Indian sauces.

FANTASTIC FOODS
1250 N. McDowell Boulevard
Petaluma, CA 94954
707-778-7801

This pioneering company produces an entire line of packaged natural foods and seasonings that take the stress out of preparing a healthy meal.

DEAN AND DELUCA, Inc.
Mail-Order Department
560 Broadway
New York, NY 10012
800-221-7714
212-431-1691

International ingredients specifically for Italian, Mexican, Chinese, Japanese, Indonesian, and Indian cooking.

NATURAL WORLD
7373 N. Scottsdale Road
Suite A-280
Scottsdale, AZ 85253
1-800-728-3388

For nontoxic and environmentally friendly home cleaning products.

Spiritual Lifestyle Support

WINGS OF SONG
Spring Hill Music
P.O. Box 800
Boulder, CO 80306

Sacred vocal music from the great spiritual traditions on CD and cassette.

BOMBAY INCENSE COMPANY
P.O. Box 915802
Longwood, FL 32791
407-699-5208
Fax: 407-869-9232

Incense and incense burners, essential oils.

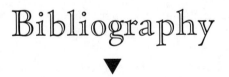

Bibliography

Achterberg, Jeanne. *Woman As Healer*. Boston: Shambala, 1990.

Atlas, Nava. *The Wholefood Catalog*. New York: Fawcett Columbine, 1988.

Benson, Herbert, M.D. *The Relaxation Response*. New York: Avon Books, 1975.

Bragg, Paul C., N.D., Ph.D., and Patricia Bragg, N.D., Ph.D. *Apple Cider Vinegar Miracle Health System*. Santa Barbara, Calif.: Health Science, 1993.

——. *Apple Cider Vinegar Miracle Health System*. Santa Barbara, Calif.: Health Science, 1995.

——. *The Miracle of Fasting*. Santa Barbara, Calif.: Health Science, 1992.

Chopra, Deepak, M.D. *Ageless Body, Timeless Mind*. New York: Harmony, 1993.

——. *Quantum Healing*. New York: Bantam, 1989.

Cichoke, Anthony J., D.C. *Enzymes and Enzyme Therapy*. New Canaan, Conn.: Keats, 1994.

Colgan, Michael, Ph.D. *The New Nutrition: Medicine for the Millennium*. Encinitas, Calif.: C.I. Publications, 1994.

Cousens, Gabriel, M.D. *Conscious Eating*. Santa Rosa, Calif.: Vision Books International, 1992.

——. *Spiritual Nutrition and the Rainbow Diet*. Boulder, Col.: Cassandra Press, 1986.

Cross, Pamela. *Kitchen Wisdom*. Ontario: Camden House, 1991.

Diamond, Harvey, and Diamond, Marilyn. *Fit For Life*. New York: Warner Books, 1985.

Diamond, Marilyn. *A New Way of Eating: From the Fit For Life Kitchen*. New York: Warner Books, 1987.

——. *The American Vegetarian Cookbook: From the Fit For Life Kitchen*. New York: Warner Books, 1990.

East-West Journal. *Shoppers Guide to Natural Foods*. Garden City Park: Avery, 1987.

Frank, Benjamin S., M.D. *Doctor Frank's No-Aging Diet*. New York: Dial Press, 1976.

Frederick, Sue, and Whiteman-Jones, Michael. *How to Shop a Natural Foods Store . . . And Why*. Boulder, Col.: New Hope Communications, 1994.

Grant, Doris, and Joice, Jean. *Food Combining for Health*. Rochester, Vt.: Healing Arts Press, 1989.

Howell, Edward, M.D. *Enzyme Nutrition*. Wayne, N.J.: Avery Publishing Group, 1985.

Kroger, William S., M.D., and Fezler, William D., Ph.D. *Hypnosis and Behavior Modification*. Philadelphia: Lippincott, 1976.

Kulvinskas, Victor P., M.S. *Don't Dine Without Enzymes*. Hot Springs, Ark.: L.O.V.E. Foods, 1994.

———. *Sprout for the Love of Everybody*. Fairfield, Iowa: 21st Century Publications, 1978.

———. *Survival Into the 21st Century*. Fairfield, Iowa: 21st Century Publications, 1975.

LaLanne, Jack. *Revitalize Your Life After Fifty*. Mamaroneck, N.Y.: Hastings House, 1995.

Lopez, D.A., M.D.; Williams, R.M., M.D., Ph.D.; and Miehlke, M., M.D. *Enzymes: The Fountain of Life*. Charleston: Neville Press, 1994.

Miles, Rosalind. *The Women's History of the World*. Topsfield, Mass.: Salem House, 1988.

Mishra, Ramurti S., M.D. *Fundamentals of Yoga*. New York: Harmony Books, 1987.

Ornish, Dean, M.D. *Eat More, Weight Less*. New York: HarperCollins, 1993.

Peale, Norman Vincent. *The Positive Principle Today*. New York: Fawcett Crest, 1976.

———. *Treasury of Joy and Enthusiasm*. New York: Fawcett Crest, 1981.

Phillips, W. Nathaniel. *Natural Supplement Review*. Golden, Col.: Mile-High Publishing, 1991.

Romano, Rita. *Dining in the Raw, Cooking with the Buff*. Proto, Italy: Prato Publications, 1993.

Santillo, Humbart, B.S., M.H. *Food Enzymes: The Missing Link to Radiant Health*. Prescott, Ariz.: Hohm Press, 1991.

Seligman, Martin E. P., Ph.D. *Learned Optimism*. New York: Simon & Schuster, 1990.

Szekely, Edmond Bordeaux. *The Book of Living Foods*. Matsqui, B.C.: I.B.S. International, 1977.

———. *The Essene Gospel of Peace, Book Four: The Teachings of the Elect*. Matsqui, B.C.: I.B.S. International, 1981.

———. *The Essene Gospel of Peace, Book Three: Lost Scrolls of the Essene Brotherhood*. Matsqui, B.C.: I.B.S. International, 1981.

———. *The Essene Gospel of Peace, Book Two: The Unknown Books of the Essenes*. Matsqui, B.C.: I.B.S. International, 1981.

———. *The Essene Science of Life*. Matsqui, B.C.: I.B.S. International, 1986.

Tourneau, Isabelle. *Cooksource*. New York: Doubleday, 1990.

Walker, N.W., D. Sc. *Fresh Vegetable and Fruit Juices*. Prescott, Ariz.: Norwalk Press, 1970.

Wheater, Caroline. *The Juicing Detox Diet*. London: Thorsons, 1993.

Wigmore, Ann. *Be Your Own Doctor*. Wayne, N.J.: Avery, 1982.

———. *Recipes for Longer Life*, Wayne, N.J.: Avery, 1978.

———. *The Sprouting Book*. Wayne, N.J.: Avery, 1986.

Woteki, Catherine E., Ph.D., R.D., and Thomas, Paul R., Ed.D., R.D. *Eat for Life*. New York: HarperPerennial, 1993.

Yogananda, Paramahansa. *Autobiography of a Yogi*. Los Angeles: Self-Realization Fellowship, 1987.

⌒⌒

IF YOU WOULD LIKE

FURTHER INFORMATION ABOUT

FITONICS™

PRODUCTS, HYPNO-MEDITATION WEIGHT-LOSS AND

RELAXATION TAPES, AND LIGHTWALKERS TRAINING

YOU CAN CALL 1-888-FITONIC

OR

VISIT US AT WWW.FITONICS.COM

⌒⌒

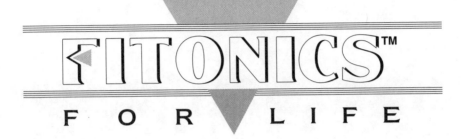

Subject Index

Recipe Index